APOCALYPSE BLUE

APOCALYPSE BLUE

MITCH GOLDMAN

Sense of Wonder Press
JAMES A. ROCK & COMPANY, PUBLISHERS
ROCKVILLE • MARYLAND

Apocalypse Blue by Mitch Goldman

SENSE OF WONDER PRESS
is an imprint of JAMES A. ROCK & CO., PUBLISHERS

Apocalypse Blue copyright ©2008 by Mitch Goldman

Special contents of this edition copyright ©2008
by James A. Rock & Co., Publishers

Address comments and inquiries to:
SENSE OF WONDER PRESS
James A. Rock & Company, Publishers
9710 Traville Gateway Drive, #305
Rockville, MD 20850
E-mail:
jrock@rockpublishing.com   lrock@rockpublishing.com

Internet URL: www.rockpublishing.com

ISBN-13/EAN: 978-1-59663-637-8

Library of Congress Control Number: 2007920282

Printed in the United States of America

First Edition: 2008

To Laura...

The great day of the Lord is near—

near and coming quickly.

That day will be a day of wrath,

A day of distress and anguish,

A day of trouble and ruin,

A day of darkness and gloom.

—Zephaniah 1:14-16

In the end the Earth will fight back.

You do know that, don't you?

—John Connigan

Book One

chapter 1

"What do you mean, he died in front of everyone?" Dean Miller asked. The doctor, about to start the day shift, stared at the sea of flowers that filled the cavernous emergency room. Then he turned back to Julie Shea. The nurse, who had just wrapped up the midnight shift, nodded as she applied her lipstick.

"This was from that code last night?" he asked incredulously.

"That's exactly what I mean," she said triumphantly. "The father of the bride, he arrested right on the dance floor, while dancing with his daughter. In front of ... *everyone.*"

Dean grimaced slightly. There were bouquets everywhere. The banquet hall had dropped them off, half in gratitude for the ER's all-out, but futile, resuscitation attempt, and half because they had no idea what to do with them, the mortified guests refusing to touch them.

He frowned at the ensemble of colors, thinking how odd it was that the same flowers could suit any occasion. The same ones that were so joyous last night now appeared solemn, almost morbidly beautiful. In the rough and tumble ER of North General Medical Center, they eerily lent a tranquil, dignified air to the place.

"It was horrible," Julie said, a hint of drama in her voice. Her eyes scanned the assembled group of incoming and outgoing ER staff. "He was only fifty and never sick a day in his life. And, then, *pow*, he went down like he'd been shot! EMS said the Best Man was doing CPR on him right by the cake. Not that it ever helps—by the time we got him in the code room he was bluer than the icing."

"The whole thing was crazy," another night nurse added. "I mean, half the wedding party was here. The men were in tuxes, the women were in these drop-dead gorgeous dresses, and the poor bride—she wore the most beautiful gown. She was so hysterical that she fainted. You know, we almost had to register her as a patient."

The two women looked at each other and nodded, satisfied that they were successfully retelling the story. The entire ER staff was mesmerized.

Dean shook his head. Fifty years old, he thought. They're getting younger and younger. Maybe it's just me, getting older and older.

"It was so sad," Julie said. "You just had to feel for that poor girl."

"The aunt, she was the tough one," the other nurse added, snapping her gum. "She held everything together. This place was going ballistic."

"The whole thing was weird," a paramedic said. "All these dressed up people walking around. The junkies didn't know whether to bow to them or start mugging them."

Another doctor, Bob Finkel, cleared his throat. "I have this to say— screw the flowers. Why didn't they drop off any Swedish meatballs?"

The entire group burst into laughter.

"You are so bad," the unit secretary said to him, smiling broadly. "Don't you have any compassion for those poor people?"

"I'm bursting with compassion. I'm dripping with compassion. All I asked for was some meatballs. And, if it will make you feel any better, I'd settle for some shrimp or little cocktail hot dogs. Hey, we're talking about wedding food. This is big stuff."

"Bad, bad, bad," Julie said with a giggle.

"Me, bad? *Moi?* All I want is just to rescue that great food. You've got a sweet tooth, I've got a fat tooth. I presume that you do know it's a waste of a cow's life to have its meatballs uneaten. Nurse, I'm trying to save a bovine soul."

"You tell me right now you don't think it's sad," the other night nurse said.

"Of course it's sad," Finkel said. "Everything is sad. We work in an ER. People don't come in for ice cream. All I'm saying is we should get some meatballs out of the deal. Remember this and do not forget—you cannot eat flowers. Get rid of them."

Julie put her finger down her throat and faked retching in Finkel's direction. The lanky doctor put down his chart, a contemplative look on his face.

"Actually, the one I really feel sorry for is the groom," he said, turning to Carol, the head nurse, who was standing a few feet away, wryly watching the proceedings. "It's not exactly conducive to the old *l'amore.* He got all dressed up, and then had nowhere to go. Know what I mean, darlin'?"

Carol seemed bemused by the whole situation. She was known for her toughness—nothing ever seemed to surprise, shock or bother her. She looked at Finkel, who was scratching a two-day's growth of beard, and smiled.

"Yeah, he didn't get nothing last night," she finally agreed. She walked over to a large grease board on a nearby wall and began writing names, matching nurses to assigned areas.

"You both are so bad," the secretary said, her eyes flashing with amusement.

"In a way I agree with Bob," Dean said. "These flowers give me the creeps. Doesn't anyone else think they're just a little weird?"

"Don't worry, hon, they're already starting to disappear," Carol said, not turning around. "People are taking them home, a few at a time."

"Maybe we should give some to the patients," Harry, a medical student, said hopefully. "It might be a nice gesture. You know, good for public relations."

Finkel put a hand on Harry's shoulder. "I'm glad that you're trying to say something smart. It represents progress. I'm almost willing to forget what you did to Bed Four yesterday. However, first let me point out that most of our patients need police, not public, relations. Second, most would try to smoke them. And finally, we don't really have to do anything, they're stealing them as we speak."

"Well, as long as they get out of here," Dean repeated.

"They're totally gross," Carol agreed, walking back to the group. "I'll call Housekeeping to dump them."

"Oh, no, they're too pretty," Julie whimpered. "Let's keep them around just for a little while longer."

She looked at Dean with a coy pout.

He looked at her, uneasy in the presence of her beauty. Suddenly, he plucked a pink flower from a nearby bouquet and put it in her hair. The entire group made approving cooing noises, except for Carol, who stole a glance at Finkel, then looked down and away. Julie stood there, beaming with delight. She re-arranged the flower in her wavy brown hair and tilted her head jauntily.

"My hero," she said.

Two ⬛⬛⬛ aides, newly hired, were walking through the area. They had been listening to the banter, their mouths half open. They had been in-serviced about their jobs, but not the subculture of the emergency room—this they would have to learn on their own. In time they would embrace it or despise it—no one could ever be neutral about working down here.

"Do they always talk like that?" one of them whispered to one of the night nurses.

"No, not really," he said. "Sometimes it gets pretty gross."

"Sometimes it … I thought ERs were serious."

"They are. And this happens to be the best in the city. If you want the politically, socially correct stuff try the reruns on Channel Three. Or come around when Administration drops by, not that they even know where this place is. "

"Okay, people, let's break it up and get to work," Carol said flatly. Unthinkingly she was running her fingers through her own hair, which was black and closely cropped. "You know the deal, save lives, wipe out disease …"

"Wait a minute," Finkel said, perplexed. "I thought we were supposed to save disease and wipe out lives. You mean, I've had it backwards all this time?"

"Yeah, Bob, I was fixing to tell you one day," Carol said dryly. "I just was waiting for the right moment."

The new employees looked at each other, their eyes wide with astonishment. Finkel eyed them dryly and casually walked in their direction. When he was certain they were within earshot he cleared his throat and turned to Julie and the other nurse who had worked with her on the "Wedding Case," as it would come to be known in the ER lore. They looked at him expectantly.

"This has gone too far, and I'll have no more of this banter," he said sternly. "This is an Emergency Room and we are to behave and talk professionally. No personal talk, now or ever. Do I make myself understood."

Julie looked at him quizzically. Finkel approached her and touched her shoulder.

"Now kiss me, baby, and get back to work."

Laughingly, she pushed him away. The nurse's station began to buzz with conversation, as doctors, nurses and aides began signing out to their replacements. Within minutes, the group started to split in half, the day and midnight shifts each going their own respective ways.

"There's a doctor call on line one," the secretary suddenly called out. "He said it's about a patient coming in."

"What else do they ever call for?" Finkel asked sarcastically. "One day one of them will call just to say, 'hello, how are you', and I'll die of a heart attack."

Dean walked over to a wall phone. "Dr. Miller." he said, absently staring at the flowers.

"Dr. Miller, my name is John Sherwin. I'm an internist down in Baltimore. I just got word that my father, George, is being taken to your hospital. My mother said it was chest pain. Could you check him out and call me back?"

"Sure, I'll watch out for him," Dean said. He scanned the electronic patient roster on the wall. "There's no one by that name in the ER. Call back in about a half hour."

The red code phone rang once. Finkel leaped up to get it.

"Thanks," Dr. Sherwin said. "He's got hypertension, diabetes and cholesterol but overall he's in pretty good shape. He retired last week. He and my mom are moving to Florida next month. They paid their dues, I'm really glad for them. "

"Hold on a second," Dean said. He cupped the receiver and looked at Finkel, who was putting a piece of gum in his mouth. This meant only one thing—Finkel was practically superstitious about some things. "What's coming in?"

"Full arrest. Seventy-year-old male. Doesn't look very good."

Dean paused, knowing the answer before he asked the question.

"How old is your father?" he asked Dr. Sherwin.

"Seventy."

Dean nodded grimly. He absently started rubbing his forehead, as if he were trying to will away any emotion.

"Hello? Doctor Miller?"

"Yeah, I'll keep a lookout. Leave your number with the secretary, Okay?"

"Thank you. Please say hello to Dad for me, and tell him that everything is going to be all right."

When Dean hung up, he could already make out the faintest trace of a siren in the distance. And that no doubt is Mr. Sherwin, he thought. He picked up a nearby white carnation, marveling at its richly textured ruffle. So what gives, he asked it silently, is this part of some cosmic blueprint, some God thing, or is Mr. Sherwin just having a really bad day. I bet you know, little flower, I bet you know everything. And while you're at it, talk to me about the father of the bride. Give me a hint—c'mon, I won't tell a soul. The approaching siren grew louder. I'd love to know, he mused, staring at the ambulance entrance, knowing that at any moment EMS would burst through, rushing their patient into the code room. And thus begins the final act of Mr. George Sherwin, he thought. Another dead person. I bet I've seen a thousand by now.

The code team was starting to assemble, dutifully taking its cues from Carol, who was placing people at strategic points around an empty stretcher. Dean wasn't technically working this area of the ER—yesterday he had walked over to the master schedule and penciled his name next to the less intense Intermediate Care Section, grateful there had been an open slot. He recognized in himself the early to middle stages of ER burnout, and after twenty years he found himself shying away from, as Finkel liked to say, all the drama and trauma. He was grateful he wouldn't have to field the inevitable return call from this man's son—let someone else tell him his father no longer existed. For Dean this was still the hardest part of his job—after all this time it was as painful as ever.

He shuffled down the hall to his assignment. People are just a bunch of moving parts assembled by God, you know, refrigerators with souls. Minor breakdowns, no sweat, we fix 'em down here, we're people mechanics. But eventually, everyone goes back to the shop, or junkyard, for that matter. It does seem like an awful lot of effort. After all is said and done, what *is* the point.

He looked at Julie, who was zipping up her jacket. She smiled at him, absently re-arranging the flower in her hair.

"Why, why, why?" he asked her.

"Why what?" she asked back, cocking her head slightly.

He just shrugged and walked away.

chapter 2

A few days later Dean rubbed his burning eyes and tried to focus on his next patient. It was almost six in the morning. He'd been working the night in Express Care.

"My foot hurts," Maximo said.

Dean looked at Maximo, otherwise known as Caveman, seated before him. He was filled with a mixture of awe and nausea. This man was practically a living legend in the ER, someone so disheveled, so derelict, so far removed from civilization as it was commonly practiced that he seemed to be of another species. It was rumored that he was one of the underground people, and had not washed in years; Finkel had once speculated that his clothes and wild beard gave hope to the endangered plant and insect species of the world- they seemed alive and well all over him.

This night has been a real loser, Dean thought bitterly. Already I've had three STDs, two impending DT's, the Human Fungus, and now, the Caveman. What crime did I commit in my last life to have deserved this? Why did he decide tonight to come out of the subway tunnels. And once I wanted more than anything to save guys like him. What's happened to me. Did I change, lose it, or just wake up.

"Ah, your foot hurts," he finally said dryly, almost painfully. "And how long have you had this symptom?"

"Three months."

"And of course you chose this night to go public," Dean said. "Could you perhaps describe in a little more depth how your foot feels?"

10

"I can't walk, and white bugs are coming out of the shoe."

"That'll do it, Max, you can stop now."

Somewhere outside of the cubicle there was the distant, muffled sound of shattering glass. Dean was exhausted. He rubbed his face and forehead with the sleeve of his white coat, looking with annoyance at the oil and dirt he had just smeared on it. For a moment he felt certain that he would vomit. The smell of this patient was unbearable.

I can't take it, I can't take it, he thought. This is not what I signed up for.

"Maximo, we're going to wash up before we do anything else. Otherwise, one of us is going to die. You come with me."

The patient was surprisingly passive. He was famous for his violent temper, but at this hour- Dean wondered if this was late night or early morning for him- he was acting like a puppy. Good for you, Mr. Caveman, Dean thought, we're gonna clean up your act.

He walked Maximo into a side room. Inside stood a giant tub that had been there for years. As always it was filled with warm water and a variety of soaps and disinfectants. It was guaranteed to kill anything. Yellow brown foamy antibiotic suds bubbled to the top.

"Hop in," Dean gestured.

"With my clothes on?" the patient asked.

"Oh yeah, I forgot. Take them off and throw 'em in the red bag over there. We'll give you new stuff. No offense, but we're gonna burn the crap you have on."

"Doc, you're the boss."

"Scrub up good," Dean said. "I'll be back."

Miller slowly got up and sidestepped out of the room, but not before seeing his patient remove what had to be the filthiest underpants he had ever seen. God, even the germs on him must be grossed out. Thank you, Max, for once again turning me off to the human race, although I must say that this been getting easier and easier lately without any help from you.

chapter 3

The tired doctor shuffled down the long, lime-colored hallway that connected the three sections of the emergency department—the main ER, nicknamed the Big Room; Intermediate Care, or Walk-In; and the dreaded Express Care Section, otherwise known as Crawl-In, depending on who was present during the conversation. Finkel said that you were really ready to be put out to pasture when you volunteered to work there. When Dean got to the end of the hallway he turned into the giant, carnival-like Big Room, once his favorite place in the world.

It was an enormous rectangle of a room, partitioned into twenty four cubicles by flimsy curtains. Each area was theoretically an independently-functioning area, equipped with anything a physician might need on the spot, including suture kits, oxygen ports, cardiac monitors, splinting materials, intubation kits, or forceps. Under ideal conditions—which usually meant immediately preceding state inspections—each area functioned as an independent treatment area.

The room was brightly, almost garishly lit. It gave one the impression of a glary day at the beach, and indeed some of the employees actually wore tinted glasses there. The staff secretly attributed their high incidence of insomnia not to the intense pressure, but to the light. Only the cigarette smokers ever glimpsed the outside world; for everyone else this was their universe, twelve hours at a time. The dominating, all-inclusive color was pale lime, which long ago had poisoned everyone's opinion towards green in general.

The place was jammed. It was a foregone conclusion that every space had a patient in it, each having waited over four hours for this privilege. Other patients rested on stretchers that seemed strewn in every available spot. Most of them were lying quietly, but several were shouting or calling for help; the one in Bed Three was bloody and screaming in pain. Miller shook his head in semi-amusement—of course this was the one patient who didn't seem to have an IV or oxygen.

Doctors and nurses ran everywhere, criss-crossing and scurrying in every conceivable direction. This was a typical shift, and the place was flooded with crises. Still, everyone moved with self-confidence and a reassuring coolness. As wild as the place seemed to be, and to be sure, at least two or three patients died in this room every day, they actually were in complete control. When Dean was hired eight years ago, Tannenbaum, his new chief, remarked to him, "You'll find that your new hero is going to be the mythological giant Antaeus. The more he was thrown to the ground, the stronger he became."

Miller relaxed as soon as he entered the Big Room, imagining himself a gladiator walking into a familiar arena. He had no work or responsibility here, having signed himself up for the lowly Express Care for the entire night shift. He had by now completely regretted his decision. He always preferred the Big Room, being completely relaxed in this bloodstained bee hive. There was nothing more enjoyable for him than to be suturing up a jaggedly torn scalp or popping a dislocated shoulder back into place. The swirling grunts, shouts, screams, beep, and bells would blend into a soothing, loud hush, much like a rumbling oceanfront. And typically, regardless of how brutal, tragic or chaotic his ER shift would be, he'd wake up the next morning, or afternoon for that matter, refreshed and remembering practically nothing of the day before.

In the very center of the room was the work station. It was a four-sided battery of desks and counters that faced outward. The desktops were lined with phones, charts, journals, newspapers, half-eaten doughnuts, and cold, long forgotten cups of coffee. In the old days they used to smoke there, too. The configuration reminded everyone of an encircled wagon train, and many times the staff did have the sensation of being surrounded by enemies.

Dean casually walked into the station, as always appreciative and secretly amazed that he was so accepted that everyone there looked up at him and just smiled. He walked over to an open chair and sat down wearily.

The midnight shift was soon ending, and the outgoing group was intensely finishing its work, trying to make things as easy as possible for the early morning reinforcements. It was considered bad form to leave too many loose ends for the new people, and unspoken was the realization that these last cases were most likely everyone's weakest, due to near suffocating fatigue—no one wanted their work scrutinized in their absence.

Miller looked around, nodding with approval. By pure chance, several of his good friends were on this night. Tannenbaum's scheduling practices could generously be called eccentric, and everyone worked different shifts all the time. Pound for pound this ER was considered one the best in the city, staffed by doctors and nurses who gave one hundred per cent of themselves each day. And the chief pretty much left them alone—the place seemed to run as if on automatic pilot. All Tannenbaum asked was that they show up on time, do a good job, and document thoroughly. There was no dress or hair code, no obligation to look "professional" and, as the saying went, there were no clocks to punch or butts to kiss. Do your absolute best, do what's right, the chief would say, and they'll know you're the real thing.

In one corner of the station sat his good friend Dan Ehler, who as usual was surrounded by half completed charts. By all accounts the hardest worker and certainly the most serious doctor on staff, Ehler had a habit of working at breakneck speed, seeing up to ten patients at a time for three, four, sometimes five hours in a row, without charting, then spending up to one hour writing them up, and tying up loose ends. It was not considered good practice—Finkel once called it playing speed chess with human pieces—but Ehler got away with it because he was so good, and no one ever complained because he always did much more than his fair share.

Next to him was Bob Finkel, arguing a case over the phone. Tall and thin, slightly graying, in need of a shave, and dressed in jeans and a ripped scrub shirt, he looked like a derelict patient half the time, but was so brilliant that no one minded. His sarcasm and cynicism were legendary. He was, nevertheless, accepted and admired by his peers, who found his work brilliant and his comments hilarious, and condoned by his superiors because they realized that he got the job done. He'd actually never been known to make a major mistake—they just don't know where to look, he would say with a sly grin. More than once he had bailed out less competent physicians. His patients loved him because he was notoriously generous with pain medications—as Finkel said, if it keeps them quiet, it keeps me happy, and on top of that, everyone from Administration down to the patient's family thinks I'm a god.

Helen Carpenter, a second year medical resident, slept in her chair in another corner. A former psychiatric nurse who had gone back to medical school, she frequently worked in the ER as an elective. All medical and surgical residents were required to spend at least one elective month per year down here, but most hated it, treating the time as little more than a prison sentence. Their relationships with the ER doctors were mostly cordial at best; for every resident who respected Dean and his colleagues as shock troops on the front lines against death, there were several more who felt them to be glorified medics—indecisive losers who couldn't get a real job.

Helen was strongly pro-ER, however, and was in the process of switching her residency to emergency medicine. She had already spoken with Tannenbaum about getting credit for her time already spent on the med-surgery floors, and then joining his department upon graduation in two years. She was already treated by everyone as one of the staff.

Many men found her to be beautiful. Dean had instantly been attracted to her, and often stole glances, haunted by her large, expressive green eyes, and her full, soft appearing mouth which hardly ever seemed to smile. Dean prided himself in being able to "read people," even after one encounter, but he just couldn't break Helen's code—sometimes she seemed mysterious, sometimes sad, but, always, many-layered. This only made her more alluring. He had never approached her, keeping his desires to himself. For one thing, he knew it was inappropriate to make an advance on a junior colleague, especially one with whom he would soon be working on a long-term basis. He had also been struggling (until a few months ago, when he just gave up), to salvage, then mourn, his failed marriage. But, mostly, it was Helen's distance, even when she seemed happy, that kept him away. It was simply impossible for him to figure out her moods, let alone her thoughts. So, Dean just let her be.

Now, she was swaying gently in her chair, sometimes jerking herself upright in her sleep, oblivious to everything. Doctors falling asleep in the midst of their comrades was an accepted tradition, proof of having worked long and hard, and "gotten the job done." No one except Dean paid her any mind.

He could have stared at her endlessly—my secret, mysterious goddess, he thought—but it seemed a little lewd, and he felt a tinge of guilt. Just as he began to reluctantly break his gaze she opened her eyes and looked at him, smiling. He turned his head awkwardly, blinking. It was like looking into the sun.

He gratefully turned to Finkel.

"Dude," Dean said, trying to sound casual.

His friend shot up a hand. "Wait," Finkel hissed, his eyebrows twisted with mischief. "I'm gonna get this guy. He forgets he's dealing with the master fisherman. Watch me reel him in." Finkel turned to the receiver.

"Listen, of course, if you don't think this admission is justified, then come on in and discharge her. It's cool, man, you just can't do it over the phone. Those are the options—accept the patient, and I'll even write some orders for you just to get her upstairs, or you can come in and send her home. Your choice, oh, and by they way, my boards are just as good as yours. In fact, I've got two boards to your one ... hey! Oh my goodness, he hung up on me!" Finkel stared at the phone, smirking.

"Sounds like you're having fun," Dean said.

"Yup," Finkel said with a grin. "I love riding this guy. The patient in question is a member of the more-toes-than-teeth crowd, some IV drug abuser with cardiomyopathy, renal failure, hep B, hep C, et cetera, et cetera. And now she's in pulmonary edema. Mark my words, this one's gonna need dialysis ..."

"And the worst part is that she smells," Carol interjected. After eighteen years in city ERs, the head nurse had become so cynical that even Finkel was impressed with her. She turned to him. "She stinks worse than my dog on a rainy day. Doesn't that bother you?" she demanded.

"I'm shocked and appalled."

"After all this time I still can't take that in a woman," she continued. "With men I expect it, they're pigs anyway."

She blew Finkel a kiss. He winked at her and resumed his presentation.

"I almost had a heart attack putting in her central line," Finkel continued. "She's hypoxic, hypotensive, pancytopenic, and has a creatinine of six. Frankly, if she were a horse I'd shoot her. Naturally, Robertson is willing to, quote, unquote, see her in his office later today, which is, of course, unacceptable to everyone except malpractice lawyers. So we're playing the game. He's trying to stall until eight o'clock, when he goes off call. For two hours he's been telling me to get one test after another—next, he'll want the broom of the wicked witch. He should have just said, thank you Dr. Finkel, and then rolled over, and gone back to bed. Instead, he's ruined his night with all these pages. I'm up anyway, and in a few minutes I'm calling him back and telling him that I'm reporting him to the chief of medicine. All this over a patient who's gonna sign herself out of the hospital in six hours. It's a joke."

"You'd really call the chief?" Ehler asked, without looking up. The doctor in question was the president of the American Board of Medicine. Even the great Tannenbaum treated this man with respect and caution.

"Of course not, but he doesn't know it, and it guarantees he'll never go back to sleep. Robertson's okay. Maybe I didn't appreciate his comments about me being 'only an ER doctor', but I've had worse. Eventually he'll come to love and cherish us—how many times have we kept guys like him out of jail from the botch-ups they made the day before. This is just a typical game on a typical night."

"Is this patient a *shpos*?" Harry asked. He has been intently listening to the interchange.

"Where'd you learn that word?" Dean asked with a half smile.

"Doctor Finkel taught it to me," the student replied proudly. "It's an acronym that stands for 'sub-human piece of shit.' Well, is she?"

"Bob, you're corrupting him already?" Carol asked. "He's just been here for two weeks."

"I've got to teach him something," Finkel answered defensively. He looked at Harry. "She's actually pretty nice, and I do wish the best for her. She's certainly made some unfortunate life choices, and they will do her in. The "S" word is reserved for special people. Doctors can be shpos, too, if you haven't already noticed."

"In Baltimore, we used to call them '*fubars,*'" Ehler said, again without looking up from his chart. "It stands for 'fucked up beyond all recognition.' Hey, the screamer just shut up. He's either a lot better or a lot worse. Who's taking care of him? Listen to how quiet it just became."

"I don't hear anything," Julie said, sipping a cup of coffee. She was seated next to Helen, who gently swayed as if dreaming. Engaged to a "consultant" who seemed to spend most of his time out of town, she was by far the most pro-doctor of all the nurses, whose relationships with the doctors ranged from romantic and outright hostility. The doctors indeed treated her like an insider, and were totally at ease with her. For Julie this caused a certain friction between her and some of her co-workers. They didn't trust her, but she couldn't care less, having long ago announced her "game plan": one day marry, move to the country, and have "as many kids as my plumbing allows."

Ehler looked up, frowning at a silent alarm that seemed to be going off in his brain.

"Something's up," he whispered, leaning forward. Shaking it off, he turned to Dean. "How you doing, guy, I haven't seen you in a few days."

"Nothing to report" Dean answered, looking around. I thought I'd be feeling better by now, he thought. "Nothing interesting going on, nothing at all. Actually, tonight has been a pain in the ass. I feel like running off to the Amazon and hiding out."

"I warned you about working in Crawl-In," Finkel mumbled, intently writing on a chart.

Dean looked in his friend's direction and glumly nodded.

"That divorce really killed him," Carol whispered to Julie, who nodded sympathetically. "Remember how sweet and cheerful he used to be?"

"I used to try to line up my shifts for when he was working," Julie whispered back. "He always used to make everyone laugh."

"People, listen to me," a dietary aide, said, pushing a cart loaded with trays past the station. "I got ten meals and there are eleven patients on this side. Who's the lucky person not getting hospital food?"

"You've got it wrong," Carol said, frowning at her clipboard. "There are ten patients and ten trays. Don't make me crazy."

"Fine with me, I'm just a dumb aide. But even though I can't count past twenty I can definitely count up to eleven. And that's how many people are in this section."

"Wait a minute. Who's in Bed Three?" Carol asked apprehensively. She stood up nervously, glancing at the half-closed curtain.

"The ambulance dropped him off about an hour ago," Harry said. "I signed for him. I thought someone told you."

"No one tells me anything. Which doctor is taking care of him?"

"Is that the screamer, by any chance?" Dean asked, knowing the answer well in advance.

Ehler looked up, frowning. "Fink, you're taking care of him, right?"

"No, I've been playing with two asthmatics, an overdose, the dislocated shoulder, and that train wreck for the past hour. I thought you or Helen were."

"No, I've been with a kidney stone, two kids and a smoke inhalation," Helen said softly, shaking the sleep from her eyes. She looked at Dean and playfully stretched. He smiled and looked down.

Ehler grimaced and looked at Carol, who shook her head disgustedly. He rose and walked over to the now silent patient.. Everyone watched him disappear behind the charcoal splattered lime green curtain. A few seconds later whipped it open to reveal a purplish, blood-soaked body. His eyes boiled with emotion.

"Call a code!" he snapped. "Get the crash cart. Let's go!"

Everyone except Dean jumped to their feet and headed for the cubicle, which belatedly started to bulge with medical personnel. As he walked by Dean, Finkel leaned down to whisper, "Do you have any idea of how many forms we'll have to fill out on this one?"

Within seconds Dean was alone in the station, watching the commotion from his seat. Somebody blew it, he thought. They forgot all about an unstable patient. If this guy croaks, Administration will be on them like flies on shit. Hopefully, he stabilizes and transfers to the ICU. Then they have the hot potato. If they can just get him out of here before nine, when the big guns arrive, no one will be the wiser.

Dean observed the proceedings, mildly curious, for a few minutes. It seemed that everyone was shouting something. He watched Finkel pull a stick of gum from his shirt pocket and slip into the cubicle. Seconds later, he heard the click of a laryngoscope blade snapping into place. They were going to intubate.

Dean smiled to himself. This guy may make it after all. At least for a few more hours, anyway. Finkel never intubates dead people. Ehler probably is putting in the central line. Oh well, I guess they'll be tied up for awhile. I can't put it off any longer. It's time to see magnificent Max again.

"Doctor Miller?"

He turned to the unit secretary.

"Doctor Robertson is on the phone. He wants to give some admitting orders. Everyone's tied up with the code, what should I do?"

Dean smiled. "Put him on hold, I think he'll wait."

Wearily getting up, cursing at the minor aches in his lower back, he waved goodbye to Helen, who stared at him dreamily from across the room. Slowly, he headed back to his area.

chapter 4

What a strange existence this is, he thought as he left the Big Room. Is the whole world this crazy? Is everything this strange and distorted? Things had to have been simpler once upon a time. We've replaced superstition with cynicism, and I don't know which is worse. In any event, this is no way to live, at least not for the long run. Maybe I should open a nice suburban practice. You know, work in a nice building. Like Robertson. You drive a nice car. Drug reps bring you lunch every day. And you don't take care of people who would rob and torture you if they met you alone in an alley. What's wrong with me, why don't I want the other stuff?

As he approached his cubicle's door Dean remembered that Maximo was still in the bathtub. Oh shit, if he drowns I'm dead, he thought in a panic. And to think I was laughing at their botch-up in the Big Room. The clipboard people are going to be all over *me*. Oh, my dear Caveman, please be alive and well. He scurried down the corridor towards the utility room. As he approached, he fantasized images of lice filled bubbles floating to the top of the water and into the air. I am doomed if this creature is dead, he thought, as he swung the door open. Dean gulped, and stared hard.

Inside, his patient smiled gaily and waved at him from the bathtub. He appeared as contented as a tourist taking a bubble bath in a luxury hotel. Aside from something that looked like excrement floating in the water, nothing seemed amiss. Dean breathed contentedly, grateful that his career was still intact. *If you weren't so ugly, I'd kiss you, darling Max.*

"Now, let's take a look at your little footsie," he said affectionately as he walked to the bathtub. "Lift up your leg."

Without a word, Maximo complied. Dean frowned. "Why didn't you take your shoe off?"

"I can't do the laces. They've been stuck in place for a few months. I guess I'm out of practice."

"You're out of practice taking your shoes off?"

"It sucks, don't it?"

"All right, just sit still, I'll do it."

Dean had to cut off the laces, which had crusted into a solid mass. He grabbed the shoe and gave it a tug. It didn't budge. Dean snarled at it. He was prepared to do anything to get this man out of his ER. He tugged and pulled and twisted it—finally he felt it wobble. Hopefully, he gathered his strength and took a deep breath. *One more yank, and this man is out of my hair,* he thought, silently cursing the cold sweat popping up on his forehead.

He pulled with all his might, and the shoe broke free. The room suddenly filled with the most unbearable stench. It took all of his will power not to run into the hall.

"No offense meant, but you must improve your hygiene," Dean scolded. "Don't you realize …"

His eyes bulged in complete horror. Maximo had no foot. There was only a pus and insect covered stump sticking out of the water. Without thinking he looked down at the shoe resting in his hands. Inside was the foot. He had pulled it off.

For the first time in his career, Dean had no idea what to say. For a brief moment he considered drowning Maximo, and dumping him and his foot in a big red bag, and running off somewhere—the Amazon never sounded so good.

"Are you in any pain?" he finally asked, incredulously.

"No, as a matter of fact I feel great," Maximo answered, unaware of what had happened. "You know, doc, you have a good bedside manner."

"Well, thank you," Dean stammered. "Listen, I just took a biopsy of your foot. I'm going to take it to the lab. Put your leg back in the water and wait here. Do not move. I want you to relax, okay?"

"Doc, anything for you."

"Take it easy now, Max, thank you. Now just stay put."

Dean eased out of the room, holding the foot behind his back. When outside, he tucked it under his arms like a football, and ran full speed into the Big Room, searching for his friends, desperate for advice. Maximo leaned back in the water, and decided to take a long, refreshing nap.

chapter 5

The well-dressed, sixtyish businessman clambered into the waiting taxi, smiling at the good luck of having an empty cab pull right in front of his office building the moment he walked out. He sat down heavily and slid over, annoyed at his wrinkling cotton suit, which dragged across the vinyl seat. Seconds later, his companion entered, a much younger man, somewhat overweight, but like his associate, expensively dressed.

"Where to?" the driver asked, not looking up from the yellow pad he was jotting entries into.

"Fifth and Fifty-third," the older man said. "Go through the park."

"You got it," the cab driver said.

The cab pulled away from the curb.

"Phillip, did you confirm the meeting next Wednesday?" the older man asked.

"It's at ten. You know, Richard, I'm really pissed. Tele-Dek went up two points yesterday. I could kick myself for having sold last week."

"There'll be other opportunities. You're going to realize that everything eventually averages out. The world is like that. Don't worry about it. And anyway, I think overall you did all right on the Tele-Dek deal."

"We both did."

They started to laugh.

The cab stopped at a light. The park was in view. The two passengers relaxed and peacefully stared out the window, completely lost in thoughts of recent and upcoming deals. The mid-morning street was remarkably empty of pedestrians and traffic.

"This is the way the city used to look thirty, forty years ago," Richard said wistfully, half to himself. "It was better back then."

"According to you, everything was," the younger man responded.

Suddenly the front and rear passenger side doors burst open and two men got in. The driver didn't move.

"Hey this cab is taken," the younger man said with annoyance.

The light turned green and the taxi sped off, heading into the park.

"I said, the cab is taken. What gives with you guys?"

"This gives," the intruder in the front seat said, pulling out a huge pistol. He waved it back and forth in their faces. Simultaneously, the man in the back seat pulled out a gun of his own. He stuck it in the mouth of the terrified younger man and smiled broadly, revealing a line of gold teeth.

"Hi, I'm Jack. Up front we have Ivan, and this is our good pilot, Diablo. Put all seats in the upright position, fasten your seat belts, and enjoy your trip," he said.

The cab raced through the park, passing the exit for Fifth Avenue.

"Go slow, my good man, there's no rush," Jack said. "Let's be law abiding and not get any tickets. We're early, anyway."

He pulled his gun out of Phillip's mouth and wiped it off on his suit jacket.

The two businessmen were paralyzed with terror and didn't move.

"By the way, don't try to open the doors," Ivan warned from the front. "They don't work from the inside. I set the children's safety catch. Okay, kids?" He guffawed. "And if you make one funny move you'll wind up in the trunk with the owner of this cab."

"That's where they're gonna wind up, anyway," Diablo joked, staring into the rear view mirror.

The three men smirked and laughed to themselves.

"Don't hurt us," Richard said, averting his eyes. "Take the money, watches, everything, we won't even look at your faces. See? We don't even know what you look like."

"Tut, tut, my man, don't be so materialistic," Jack admonished. His licked his lips and smiled impishly. "There's more to life than money."

"Please don't hurt us," Phillip said softly.

"Are we nervous?" the gunman asked with deeply affected concern. "Gentlemen, *ignit aurum probat.* That's Latin for, "fire tests gold." In other words, be cool, the good times don't test your character, the bad times do. And these are the bad times. So, gentlemen, let's see what you're made of. Come on, tell me your philosophy. "

"Jack, cut that shit," Diablo said. "Save it for later."

"Maybe he's right," Ivan whined. "We're almost there."

"Then just play the radio and don't listen," Jack snapped. "These are high-class people and I'm in the mood for a high-class chat."

He cleared his throat.

"Let's have a talk, you know, guy talk, heart to heart talk. Think about your lives, talk about 'em, sum 'em up, say whatever. Talk to me. My gift to you today is that of closure—that's a real break, and it doesn't happen often. It didn't happen to my daddy—he never knew what hit him. You guys should be grateful."

"Sick, sick, sick," Diablo mumbled.

"I got kids," the younger man begged, visibly shaking.

"We all got kids. You fucked someone, she got pregnant, and you want points for that?" Jack said impatiently. "Old timer, tell me about your life. Come on, entertain me."

For the next ten minutes the cab meandered through the park, while the two hostages alternately pleaded for their lives and spoke about them, hoping against hope for a reprieve. Initially, Diablo and Ivan tried to ignore the goings on, but soon found themselves hanging on every word, sometimes snickering, and sometimes nodding their heads, as if impressed by what the two men had to say.

Finally, the cab left the park and made its way into one of the more desolate parts of the city. When it finally pulled up to what seemed an abandoned garage, no one on the street looked up. A giant metal door lifted, and the garage seemed to swallow them up as they entered. The door closed.

chapter 6

The cab eased to the middle of the empty floor. The room was gray and quiet.

"Everybody, out," Jack commanded.

"Don't hurt us, please," Phillip whimpered. "I got kids."

"Fuck you and fuck your kids," Jack snarled. "Hurry up and get out. Go over to that canvas on the floor and stand on it."

Doing as they were told, the prisoners shuffled towards the center of the room, onto a huge tarpaulin. They waited nervously, looking around. Both of them saw the nearby group of men at once, standing alongside a wall, their arms folded. Diablo walked over to them and melted into their midst.

The other two men looked toward the group, smiling broadly.

"We did it, Killer, we did it, just like you wanted," Ivan said.

The man in the center of the group nodded his approval, his face bathed in shadows. He stood nearly one head taller than the other men, and his silhouette connoted a giant physique, bulging with muscles. It was obvious at once that he was the leader.

"Goody, goody for you," Killer said with a soft sarcasm. "Now do your thing."

"Yes, sir," Ivan said respectfully. He and Jack faced their two victims and donned thin leather gloves.

"Please," Phillip said softly.

"One, two, three," each counted out loud, and suddenly the attack began.

With all their might, marshaling all their stamina, they attacked their terrified victims. Each was a seasoned street fighter and their blows landed with pinpoint accuracy. The victims cowered, overwhelmed with fear and confusion. Phillip soon dropped to his knees, bellowing wildly, but Richard cursed and actually started fighting back, knocking Ivan down with a vicious hook. This elicited wild applause and derisive hoots in the audience. Ivan arose, furious at his humiliation. He landed a barrage of blows that landed with sickening thuds. The older man's knees wobbled, and he too fell to the ground.

The assault continued until both victims were lying in crumpled heaps, nearly unrecognizable.

The attacker straightened and looked up at the group. They were panting and dripping with sweat.

"Good work," Killer said casually.

The rest of the group stood impassively.

"Congratulations, you're in the Death Masters," the leader said.

The small group broke into polite applause.

"Now that you've left the other world, you belong to ours," he continued, knowing the ritual by heart. "Blah, blah, blah … shit, I been doing this way too long. Let's get it done with."

Killer unfolded his massive arms and walked over to the new gang members. They lowered their heads respectfully.

"Jack, you did okay. I think that fat boy died half-way into the beating. It's gonna be fun seeing you in action."

"Thank you, sir."

"And you, lover boy," Killer said, looking at Ivan with a hint of contempt. "You looked positively cute out there. That old guy, he hit you good. If he was ten years younger he'd have beat the shit out of you, and he'd be in the gang now."

There was a snicker in the group.

"Shut the fuck up, whoever did that," Killer said quietly, without turning around. He never took his eyes off Ivan. "You got a problem with that?"

"No, sir."

"Good, because I'm getting bored. Man, in my day we sure were a lot better with our hands. Lover boy, get rid of the bodies. Take off their clothes and burn them. Put these two gentlemen in the trunk with the driver and drop everything off at the hot dog plant. Jack, say hello to your new brothers, and then come back to the club and help yourself to whatever. Both of you, listen up, you're like trainees now. You be in my office at nine tomorrow morning. There's a lot to learn. Don't find out the hard way what happens when someone's late for a meeting with me."

With that the group walked up to the new inductees, shaking their hands and introducing themselves. Killer watched with detached amusement his thirty or so men, each fearsome in appearance, making small talk with the new members. Suddenly he snapped his fingers and signaled with his head. With that, the entire group made its way out of the garage's rear entrance.

Ivan was alone with the bodies. He cursed his luck.

Damn, I always get the shit, he thought.

Grumbling to himself, he started piling the bodies neatly on the canvas, occasionally kicking them in anger. Everybody's having fun but me, he said to himself.

He fumbled with the heavy loads, annoyed at the blood stains he was accumulating on his shirt. Then, as he was folding the bodies into the canvas, he stopped and looked around. He had heard a noise coming out of the darkness.

He perceived the faintest of motions, and he whirled around, coming face to face with two small, quiet men. He started, very upset that anyone had witnessed this episode. Something about them was unsettling, something alien and remote. Possibly it was just the way they stood and stared at him, in absolute stillness.

He realized that they weren't afraid of him, and this threw him off badly. He also sensed that they had come for him. He had no experience being a victim, and for the first time in years was afraid. Backtracking, fumbling for the gun he had always carried, he realized in his panic that his hands were shaking too much to use it effectively. All he now wanted to do was to get away from these strange people.

They moved towards him and he jumped back, tripping over the bodies. He hit the ground hard, stunned. Looking up he saw them standing over him, a faraway look in their eyes. At that moment there was a burning stab of pain on his face, and he covered it with his hands.

Within seconds he was writhing in agony, and then, suddenly, he lost all power. He lay helplessly on the ground unable to speak, unable to beg for his life, feeling as if he weighed a million pounds, and that a million more was lying on his chest. He felt his hot urine drip down his leg. His mind consumed with uncontrollable terror, he began to suffocate in silence.

The two men pounced on Ivan, tying his arms and feet. One ran over to the garage door and pulled it open. A van pulled inside. Quietly, the driver got out and walked over to inspect the catch.

"Good work," he said. "Jungle Man wants him in cage six."

Easily, the three men hoisted their flaccid victim and dumped him in the van's rear. They got into the van, and it sped off into the night. There were no witnesses.

chapter 7

A few days later, Bob McElvoy shuffled into Dean's cubicle and sat down slowly. He had waited four hours in the ER exclusively to see Dean, who he considered his private physician. Their relationship stretched back to Dean's residency days, from his clinic rotation, and they knew each other well.

When Dean saw the middle-aged man, he held his breath and smiled tightly, noting that he had lost even more weight. Two months ago, while looking at a routine chest X-ray, he had discovered a mass. Eventually a diagnostic workup revealed wildly metastatic carcinoma.

Both of them had been very upset at the way in which Bob had been told. He had been sitting in the Oncology Clinic's waiting room, worrying about the outcome of his tests, when a group of doctors walked out, followed by residents and medical students. One of the senior doctors turned to the others and said, "Listen up, this is a good teaching case." And then he turned to Bob and said, "Hi, we're the tumor doctors and you have a tumor."

From that moment, Bob was never the same. He had described it to Dean as if his insides had turned into ice, and he seemed unable to ever look up at the sky again.

Dean was angry at himself for his reaction to Bob's illness. He started avoiding him, at one point calling in sick on a day they had agreed to meet. He distanced himself emotionally from Bob when they did, keeping their meetings cool and very clinical. They had once been very close;

Bob would often show Dean photos of his recent vacations and bring cookies that his wife had baked. For his part Dean would sometimes spend up to an hour with him. He considered the slightly older man a friend, one of the very few he had.

Truthfully, Dean had entered emergency medicine because there had to be no relationships with people. What he did was pure science— a patient presented with certain signs and symptoms, and from this a diagnosis, and therapeutic plan, had to be fashioned, free of psychological or historical baggage. He rationalized to himself that this was the direction medicine was heading anyway and that he was simply ahead of his time. For him medicine was as impersonal as the board exams he had sat for, only here one dealt with living people.

On a deeper level he knew that he had difficulties with his feelings, of not wanting to touch or be touched. Awkward since childhood with his emotions, he had erected a transparent but impenetrable wall when dealing with people—Dean was the first to admit that this had probably ruined his marriage. He actually liked his patients very much, but found his distance advantageous, because he saw so much suffering every day. For him, dying and disease were the norm; you see someone bleed to death in front of you, and then you have a cup of coffee.

Things sometimes bothered him: a pregnant woman shot in the stomach, a boy with his face burned off, or a middle-aged man stroking out, forever paralyzed and speechless. And then, as always, he'd have some lunch, forget everything, and start again.

His first reaction to Bob's cancer was one of betrayal, as if Bob was some type of Trojan horse he had permitted to enter his icy fortress. He knew this was illogical and immature but he could do nothing about it.

Bob looked at him sadly. He had the air of surrender about him, of hurt and bafflement, the look of someone who had just been slapped.

"How are you feeling, Bob?" Dean asked cautiously.

"Like it's Sunday night, and I'm looking at the worst week of my life. How are you?"

"All right."

"You know, I'm a vegetarian," McElvoy blurted out. "This isn't supposed to happen to health nuts."

"It can happen to anyone," Dean said quietly, looking down and pretending to read Bob's old chart.

"I drink bottled water. I don't even smoke. Can't you do something? Please."

"There's chemotherapy. It's going to help."

"It's going to prolong, that's what it's going to do."

You're right, thought Dean. Sorry, Bob, we don't cheat death, we just stall it. We doctors have marketed this illusion that we're special. It's probably our greatest success. I'm glad you're not buying it.

"You know, Doc, I just retired."

Dean stared at Bob's muscular body, avoiding his eyes. He looked at a faded forearm tattoo, from his patient's Navy days. It was of a semi-naked hula dancer, who once moved about suggestively with various wrist maneuvers. Now she was no more than a faded shadow.

He had once seen a picture of Bob in his youthful prime. The man was standing on a dock with his wife, a beautiful woman with long, black hair and bright red lipstick. Bob was rippling with muscles and had the whitest teeth and the widest smile, and his hair was wavy and smartly combed. Dean imagined from the way they held onto each other that they had just had sex; both looked so happy.

Bob had been widowed three years. He still had the look of a puppy whose litter-mates had been sold and taken away.

"What if I drink herbal tea? I'll just clean out my system."

"I don't think that's been shown to help," the doctor said quietly, wishing his patient would somehow disappear.

"What will? Do I have any real options?"

Dean said nothing, looking down. Bob was shrinking in front of his eyes, ceasing to be a real person, becoming just another terminal unit on some cosmic loading dock, waiting to be shipped off. He didn't want to see Bob go away. God, this hurts too much, he thought. I wish I was stronger. I wish I could find some perspective to put this all in. I wish I knew how to deal with death, and life, in some way other than total withdrawal.

Dean thought of Finkel's saying, "Doctors, just like hookers, should never come with their tricks." He knew he had been attracted to the ER because of its anonymity. One never got close to a patient, and you could do and say exactly what had to be done, with no shyness and no reservations. For nearly twenty years Dean had practiced his best medicine, and it was good medicine, on people who never even inquired his name.

Why are you going to die, he thought, silently staring at his patient's shoes. I'll turn around next year and you'll be gone. All that's going to be left of you is a fat manila chart filed away in some warehouse. And when I think of you I'll miss you, you fucking traitor.

"I'll go upstate to my sister's farm," the man begged, frightened by Dean's abandonment.

"Look, I can't predict the future. But I've got connections with Oncology. I'll get you on this new test drug—it's been shown to be of benefit, or it may be that the drug reps are doing a super job of buying us pizza . I really don't know, and I am so sorry that I really don't know. Here, take this slip to the front desk and they'll set you up."

Dean held up a pink sheet of paper and held it up, still avoiding his eyes. He was filled with self-loathing. Don't take it, he wanted to scream. Run out of here and climb your last mountain. Don't let them take your dignity and hair away on this longest of shots. The extra hundred days aren't worth it.

"I can't believe this is happening to me."

"We'll see what happens, we'll see. Listen, I'm running behind with other patients. Keep me informed as to what happens. Okay?"

Bob seemed to melt before him. "I'm sorry I bothered you, Doc. I am sorry."

He slowly stood up. Dean noticed that he didn't stretch this time, as he normally did. He seemed smaller for some reason.

Dean closed his eyes. Don't come with the tricks, he kept saying, don't come with the tricks.

Against his will a small bit of sadness trickled in. Dean shook his head and silently acquiesced, letting it grow into a flood of emotions. He was going to miss Bob very much.

"Bob, let me say something. I'm not good at this kind of thing, not good at all. In fact, I'm terrible at it. It's my problem, not yours. In a lot of ways I am a very second-rate person. And, God, I'm sorry for you. In twenty years, ten years, five years, or even tomorrow I'll be in your shoes, and I won't have anything near the great life you've had to show for it. Please forgive me, and please keep your appointment. Take care of yourself."

Bob looked at his doctor and nodded.

"You got it, Doc."

He started to leave the room. Dean sat there, his face twisted with emotion. Suddenly he bolted up and faced his patient. They looked deeply into each other's eyes for a few seconds, and then reached out and hugged tightly, each feeling and accepting the other's pain.

"I'm sorry I can't cure you," Dean whispered, his eyes welling with tears.

"I know you are," Bob said. "In a way I feel worse for you."

They released their grip and stared at each other. Both had tears in their eyes.

"How long do I really have?" Bob asked through clenched teeth.

"A few months, a year. I don't know exactly. The cancer's in your liver and bones. It's a crap shoot. How strong your system is, how strong your will is, whether or not you go on chemo. What's going to happen is going to happen. Bob, these bodies of ours are rentals. We don't own them, and we certainly don't have the final say about them."

"Doc, it's a strange feeling knowing you're not going to last forever. I always felt like I was the center of the universe, and that if I were to die, everything would stop."

"Who knows, maybe it will," Dean said, forcing a smile.

"No, you'll all stick around. It won't be that bad, I guess. Can I tell you something? I know that you're busy ..."

"No, that was just an excuse. Tell me."

"When my wife Martha was dying, with her last words she asked me if I would marry her in heaven when I joined her, would I spend eternity with her. I said yes, and I meant it. So I suppose it's not all that bad. I've already got a date lined up when I get there."

They shook hands and Bob walked out, the clinic slip in his hands. Dean stood very still in the small room, thinking about life and death and love. Who knows, he thought, there just might be some hope for the world, and me, after all.

chapter 8

The overdose lay motionless on the stretcher. His face was muddied with regurgitated charcoal, which had been pumped into his stomach during the resuscitation effort. A long plastic breathing tube snaked from a respirator through his left nostril and into his lungs. Another tube had been inserted into the other nostril and threaded into his stomach. Still another went through his penis and into his bladder. His arms, legs and chest were tightly tied down.

Quietly, a figure padded into the room and approached the body. They were alone. She knelt over and deftly began to remove his rings. As with most OD victims, his other possessions had been stolen from him at the scene long before the ambulance had even arrived. She didn't realize it, but her motions had attracted attention, and someone entered the room after her.

She completed her task and began to back out of the room. Just as she turned around, she bumped into Dean, who stood before her, his arms folded.

"Gloria, how are you?" he asked with affected tenderness and concern.

"Fine, just fine," she stammered. "They paged Housekeeping to the ER, and I thought I would start in this room."

"You know, Gloria, I think something accidentally dropped in one of your pockets."

"I didn't do anything."

"I know you didn't. Like I said, what happened was an accident. These things happen. Hard to believe, isn't it."

"There's nothing in my pockets."

"Gee, Gloria, I think there is. And you know something, I believe in your complete innocence. But, let's take a look. You're going to laugh when you see the stuff in your pockets."

"Don't you touch me. I know you people."

The woman backed away, her hands rising defensively

"Gloria, I wouldn't dream of impinging on your rights. But let me call the nursing supervisor and Security. I'm sure they're going to get a good chuckle out of this. We all could use a good chuckle, right?"

He turned around and began to wave at the supervisor, who was standing nearby reviewing a chart with an administrator, when he heard some clanging on the ground. He looked down and saw the missing jewelry. Gloria glared at him with hatred.

"I knew you'd see the light. Thank you, Gloria."

She whirled around and stormed away. Dean smiled, bent down, and recovered the jewelry. After admiring it for a second, he dropped it in his lab coat and left the room, looking for the security guard known as Mr. Natural. Spotting the huge man, he walked up and gave him the items.

"Register these, they belong to the OD."

"Doc, it's good to see an honest man these days," the guard said with a smile. "You give hope to the world." He left for the security office.

Dean went back to the work station. Finkel was there, working on a sudoko puzzle. When Dean recounted what had just happened Finkel laughed heartily, not taking his eyes off the numbers.

"It's amazing," Dean said. "She commits a crime, she betrays a patient trust, she lies, and then she has the nerve to be angry with me. I can't believe some people."

"Hey, hire a shpos, you get a shpos. I lowered all my expectations about that one long ago."

"I don't need this crap. You know, yesterday I had to tell my favorite patient that he's going to die from his cancer. Remember Bob McElvoy?"

Finkel put down his puzzle and looked up. "McElvoy?" he asked softly. "You and I had him when we were residents. Oh damn, I'm sorry."

"Yeah. You want to break for some lunch?" Dean asked hopefully.

"I'd love to, but I can't. I shouldn't even be doing this puzzle but I almost got the whole thing. There's some trauma coming in. Hey, you remember your friend Magnificent Max? Well, he's up on Rehab now and seems to have fallen in love. Last night he stuck his prosthetic foot up someone's ass. Man, you've got to see that X-ray. They're framing it up in Radiology."

They shared a good laugh, and then went back to work.

chapter 9

Mr. Natural popped some pumpkin seeds into his mouth and motioned to the elderly couple standing before him.

"X-ray, huh, yeah, it's right down the hall," he drawled. With a huge hand he brushed his thinning, shoulder-length hair from his face. "You go down to the big desk and show them this here slip and they'll take good care of you."

After the couple left, Mr. Natural ate a few more seeds. He was always watching his weight and long ago had decided that pumpkin seeds were the best snack around, since so much effort and time went into retrieving so little food. With time he had evolved to the point where he now ate them nearly continuously, and when nervous, was known to chew and swallow them whole.

Standing in the dead center of the Big Room, the guard now assumed his favorite pose, hands in both rear pockets, rocking back and forth on his heels, his big belly thrust forward and his eyes closed. He began chanting softly.

A nearby group of medical residents, rotating through the ER, looked at him with contempt. They pretty much stayed to themselves, and were counting down the days to when they could return upstairs and leave this alien, sometimes hostile, world. One of the senior residents shook her head. She turned to her team, who the ER referred to not by their names but by their rank in their respective programs.

"Our In-Security guard," she said, not taking her eyes off him. "Don't you just feel so, how can I say it, safe, around him?"

"The last of the hippies," a second year added. "It's like being the last of the dinosaurs. I wonder what he thinks about."

"I just wonder if he thinks at all. That pothead just never grew up."

"A bomb could go off and he wouldn't notice," another second year said. "How can anyone be so mellow? Or should I say, oblivious."

"Massive drug abuse in your formative years will do it every time," the senior said. "You should hear the way he describes it. He's the only person I know who still brags about getting high. I don't know anyone who even admits to it anymore. He was talking once about his five hundredth acid trip. It was a big thing in his commune. They had this major ceremony, and they sent him into the woods with a backpack and all. A real religious thing."

"Well, I hope he found God that day, because I bet now he has trouble finding his way out of the bathroom."

"Just look at him, swaying out there."

"What a waste," the intern piped in. "Did you know that he lives in a glorified shack with a bunch of illegal immigrants. They pray to jungle gods and eat rice and beans every day."

"To think he went to college—yeah, he told me that. Pre-med. What a waste of a life."

They stared at the big man. His lips were moving; otherwise he was practically motionless.

"Last week he came in, I swear, half-stoned, and I got on his case. He had the nerve to get angry," the senior added defensively. "He said he was on a crusade to save the world from people like me, and that my days were numbered. What a fucker, I almost wrote him up."

"Excuse me! Don't you all have something better to do than talk about someone behind his back?" Finkel demanded, having burst in on this conversation behind them. He glared at them, noting with silent satisfaction how they nervously avoided his eyes. "Nothing better, little shits? You certainly don't have much to say when it comes to patient care—frankly, it's because I don't think any of you knows all that much. Maybe you're allergic to sick people. You certainly avoid them like, shall we say, the plague? Well, I have an assignment for you brats. We'll meet here at the end of your shift. You will present to me and anyone else who's interested, in their entirety, hallucinogens and their toxicology. Mechanisms, workups, treatments, et cetera et cetera. Try learning something for a change. So far, none of you have even come close to earning this arrogance of yours."

Finkel's eyes bored into to the residents, who began to shift uneasily.

"My mother's on the hospital's board of directors," the senior resident blurted out, in a voice mixed with defiance and mild trepidation.

"I'm sorry, am I supposed to be impressed?" Finkel asked with mock innocence.

"Her name is Susan Anderson," the resident said, his voice wavering slightly.

"And I'm sure she's the reason you got into this residency program," Finkel replied coldly, not breaking his icy stare. The resident visibly buckled under the withering gaze. The other residents cowered slightly, their leader having collapsed before their eyes.

"Two things, *Doctor* Anderson. Go call mommy. If she's half the person I think she is, then she'll be apologizing to me on your behalf. Second, I'm so sorry that you're slumming. Don't worry, it'll wash off. Fuck this assignment up, by the way, and I guarantee you'll be repeating your ER rotation, and that would be a fate worse than death, wouldn't it? Now run off to the library, you were going to sneak out of here anyway."

Finkel watched them scurry away. He shook his head. Darting his eyes at Mr. Natural, he turned and walked away, and headed for a patient's room.

They never knew it, no one ever did, but in this ER, where curtains gave the pretense of walls, everyone always seemed to speak a little too loudly, and as always, Mr. Natural heard everything. Without opening his eyes, he smiled slightly. It shouldn't be too long, not too long at all, fellas. And then, you're gonna get yours. All of you.

chapter 10

The following evening, while writing up a case, Dean broke into a clammy sweat. Instinctively, he rubbed his belly. Oh shit, cramps are on the way, he thought. He rubbed and rubbed, to no avail. Within seconds some virus or toxin or combination thereof began to wring his insides as if they were a wet towel. The only thing that would relieve the onrushing pain would be a very quick trip to the bathroom.

He motioned to Finkel and Ehler that he would be back. They nodded to him sympathetically. Dean flew out of the station, heading towards what the insiders all called 'the magic bathroom', a shockingly clean, normal place free of graffiti or marijuana smoke. Only a few staff members even knew of its presence.

After he emerged, no longer in pain but feeling drained and cold, Dean decided he wasn't in shape for a killer session in the Big Room. Too sick, he thought. Infused as he was with the code of the emergency room doctor—you can work or you can be dead, no other options—going home never crossed his mind. So, reluctantly, he picked up a house phone and called Express Care. He was connected to Helen Carpenter.

"Helen, it's Dean."

"What's the matter with you? You sound strange."

"I'm dying. Worst case of the runs I've ever had. Do me a big favor. Switch with me. You take the Big Room. Ehler is there so he can supervise your cases, not that you need it anyway. I'll finish up back where you are."

"But, Dean, you hate it here."

"Not now. At this moment Express beckons to me like a distant oasis in the desert."

"Dean, I'm sure they'll let you go home. Why don't you just take it easy?"

"Helen, please, help me out. I'd like to finish the shift. It's not right to everyone else if I go. It's just that I can't guarantee standing in any one spot for more than twenty minutes at a time, and that's not cool when you're running a code."

"Oh, Dean, you're so dedicated. Yeah, come on over. I'll wrap up what I have so I won't even have any sign-outs."

Even as sick as he was, he found himself attracted to her. He found her so very beautiful, in a special, private way, and her voice as always resonated into the very depths of his being—it was if she were talking directly to his soul. God, I'd get off my deathbed and make love to her, he thought, and then I'd go back and die, and I wouldn't even mind. She is right, I should go home. But I've never wasted a sick day on really being sick and I'm not going to start now. Besides, someone in this place gave me this bug, and damn it, I'm going to get my revenge and spread it around.

As he left the Big Room, he glanced up at the wall and smiled at the large clock, broken as it usually was. Finkel said it summed up their life in the ER, timeless and perfectly correct maybe twice a day. He went down another hallway and entered Express Care. Many doctors liked it here because it was easy—usually one neither cured nor killed in this area. The Big Room was more like a battle zone, with split second life and death decisions, and once you made that decision there was often no time to take it back, it was all or nothing. In Express one could indulge in luxuries such as eating lunch sitting down, making a personal phone call, or going to the bathroom at will. Their chief, Tannenbaum, had long ago carved out this area for both timely patient care efficiency, and for it to be some sort of safety valve for his overworked, underpaid doctors. Most found this work boring and tedious, and when they requested to work here, it usually meant they needed to take it easy.

Dean walked through Intermediate, mindlessly looking at the new, old and ancient stains that seemed to dance with each other on the cracked floor. He passed through the waiting area, nodding at the night staff, avoiding the demanding stares of the forty or so patients sitting on folding chairs in the waiting area. He ignored them for their own sake—like waiters, doctors and nurses could be quite passive aggressive. The more they were stared at, the slower they would become.

After a few pleasantries with the nurses he walked down a small corridor, noting with mild amusement that he would be working in the same room where he had seen Maximo. Maybe that bugger gave it to me, he thought, he's a walking micro lab. Well, maybe not exactly walking anymore. He removed his jacket and tossed his stethoscope onto the small desk alongside a wall. He sat down in a folding chair and rubbed his belly.

Dean did not want to be here—there was too much time to daydream. Years ago, in his old days, he'd spent chunks of his Express shift speaking with his ex-wife. Now that she was gone—or more precisely, now that she had left him, leaving him depressed and hurt—there was nothing to do here but actually work.

For the millionth time he found himself asking, why did she leave me, why'd she do it? I'd have toughed it out, why couldn't she. Was it really that bad, was I really that boring ...

"Hey, Doc."

Dean violently startled. He looked up to see Mr. Natural's smiling face.

"You okay?" the guard asked. Dean couldn't be sure if the look on the man's face was that of amusement or vague hostility.

"Yeah, yeah, sure. I was just relaxing. What's up?"

Dean looked intently at him, secretly glad to have had his thoughts interrupted.

"You're relaxing. That's good. You gotta stay loose in this place, otherwise you start to burn out."

"Sure. Did you need me for something?"

"Yeah, I need a favor. A friend of mine's in a lot of pain. I thought the lady doctor was here, but you'll do just fine."

"We switched places. Do fine for what?"

"Don't you worry, he'll love you. Can you see him out of turn? I wouldn't ask most of the other doctors, they got such tight asses when they fart only a dog could hear it. But you're a regular guy. Doc, I'd appreciate it."

Dean couldn't help but smile, taking the remark as a compliment. Unlike most of his colleagues he had not gone from high school through residency as if shot out through a tunnel. He'd gone through several jobs—once he'd even worked part time as a security guard in this very same hospital- starting medical school at age twenty-seven. While his eclectic background made him somewhat different from the other doctors who knew only one career and one perspective, he got along that much better with people from outside the profession. Almost by coincidence he'd decided one day to try out for medical school. If but for fate, he would often think while examining a patient, there go I.

Seventeen years and approximately seventy thousand patients later, he sat there looking at Mr. Natural, staring into his wide face, with its pale, saucer-like eyes.

"You got it," he said. "Bring him on."

The security guard gave him a thumb's up sign and spoke with someone apparently standing nearby.

"Come on, he'll see you now."

He tugged, and soon an arm came into view.

"Doc, I want you to meet Professor John Connigan."

He hauled his friend into the open doorway. Dean's eyes widened. Connigan was large but, unlike Mr. Natural, who had a beefy, powerful presence, he was round and fat, with puffy cheeks and an enormous pot belly. He gave the impression of complete softness and, combined with his pasty color, Dean's first impression was that the man was little more than a large mass of butter.

Although clean shaven, the man was totally disheveled, wearing dirty, grease-stained rags. His shoes were torn and mud-caked. Most unsettling, however, were his eyes. Dean's clinical skills had developed to the point where he could often make a diagnosis simply by looking at a patient, and he could do it here. There was no mistaking it. This man was insane.

"Hello, I'm pleased to meet you," Dean said, reluctantly extending a hand to his new patient, purely out of courtesy to the security guard. He slightly grimaced at the other man's cool, flaccid grip.

He looked up at Mr. Natural.

"He's your friend" he asked the guard quizzically.

"Doc, I know he don't look it, but John here is a genius, one of the greatest minds that's ever been. He's just been out of it for a few days, and I guess he looks a little frazzled. I'll take him home later. John, what do you have to say to the doctor?"

Connigan looked at Dean, who involuntarily flinched, and in a toneless voice he spoke for the first time.

"Life is like Jupiter. It's a roller coaster ride through purple infinity."

Dean looked at him for a second and snorted. He turned and looked dubiously at the security guard, who was frowning at the man.

"Natch, are we going to have any problems here?"

The guard leaned over and whispered something to his friend. It had an almost electric effect—Connigan instantly became alert. He straightened up and looked at Dean. His eyes seemed to be almost burning with forced intensity.

"So, let's begin," Dean said, uneasily. "Now, Mr. Connigan …"

"Professor Connigan," the man corrected.

"Okay, Professor Connigan. Please have a seat. Mr. Natural, I'll take good care of him."

"Thanks, Doc, I appreciate it. Here's his chart, everything's square. I'll leave you two alone now. John, you be good."

He left. Dean was alone with Connigan.

chapter 11

Because he sensed that Connigan posed no physical threat, and out of need to maintain privacy, Dean reached over and swung the door closed. Within seconds he regretted his decision—the small room filled with rancid odors. So this is his 'friend', he thought grimly. God, maybe everyone is right about Natural, maybe he does have a fried brain. Okay, we're gonna make this a quickie.

He turned in his chair to fully face his patient, who was sitting in a small metal folding chair alongside the desk. It was hard not to feel repulsion for the man, who continually wiped his dirt encrusted hands through his short blonde hair. Mucous was running freely from both nostrils, which he seemed to ignore. He held a small book.

"So, Professor, what can I do for you?"

"An apocalypse in blue approaches. It will sweeten our world, and caress us as we sleep. We will wake up to a new dawn."

"Excuse me?"

"You can stop it, you know, you can block everything," the ragged man mumbled. He slumped in his chair and started to drift off.

And I hope you go to hell for bothering me in the middle of the night, Dean wanted to say. He felt the slightest rumble of thunder in his belly. Not again, he thought. I just got the two minute warning.

Fighting against his pain, he decided to quickly determine if this man was really a professional, to be treated as something of an equal, or merely a delusional mental patient with a vivid imagination.

48

"Listen, wake up and talk properly. I want appropriate answers or you'll go to the waiting room and wait for your rightful turn. I don't have the time or inclination to deal with nonsense. Do you hear me?"

Connigan actually seemed to respond. He nodded, looking at the ground sadly. Dean got the sense the man was trying with all his might to concentrate. He felt remorseful at having spoken so roughly. "Are you really a professor?"

"Viral genetics, from Princeton. I don't come off like one, do I?"

"It's okay. I don't come off like a doctor."

Dean paused, thinking back to his university days. His favorite subject had been genetics—once he'd even considered teaching it for a career. Let's see if he's legit, he thought. He squinted and tapped his chin, thinking of what to say.

"What's the genetic mechanism of damage caused by ultraviolet radiation?"

Connigan looked up at him. "Thymine dimerization, secondary to covalent bonding by a cyclobutan ring. It shuts down DNA replication."

"Okay. Uh, what are the four stages of polypeptide chain synthesis?"

"Activation, initiation, elongation, and termination. Activation, by the way, takes place in the cytoplasm, where the amino acids are bound to their corresponding RNA via esterifacation. I didn't know if that was going to be your next question."

"I'm sorry, I'm sorry," Dean said, slightly flustered. Then he caught himself, and said indignantly, "Hey, listen, you don't exactly look like a scientist. I think you know what I mean."

"Once I did. Things just didn't work out as planned," Connigan said through clenched teeth, clearly in pain. "Once I thought things would all fall into place; instead, they fell on me."

For a brief moment, Dean had been taken aback by a flash in Connigan's eyes. But just as he was about to start consoling the disheveled man, Connigan looked at the ceiling and exhaled deeply. Dean got the distinct impression of a man who had just slipped away.

Dean didn't know what to think. This man was certainly was not a typical street person. His education was apparent, his answers revealing a causal brilliance. He studied the man for a few seconds, when he was interrupted by a small cramp. He snapped into action.

"Professor, what can I do for you?"

"Pain. In my head. My brain is on fire. I was shot in the head a few years ago. I get bad headaches. Sometimes I can get into the pain; sometimes I can ignore it. But it's bad now, and I can't do my work. All I do now is cry and retch. I can't take it any more. And I've got to finish my work."

"What work," Dean asked skeptically.

"I'm going to save the world. Thanks to lac operon."

"*Lac operon*? As in microbiology? What does that have to do with …"

"Give me something for the pain," Connigan whispered urgently.

Another cramp hit Dean, this one more powerful than the rest. I can't hold out much longer, he thought.

"Listen, Professor, I'm in a rush. I'm going to examine you. If I think there's something I can do for you, than by all means I'll prescribe some hydrocodone …"

"Morphine."

"What did you say?"

"I want injectable morphine, twenty milligrams, IV push. And add twenty-five of diphenhydramine to the solution."

Ah, so that's your game, Dean thought, disappointed in the man. He was angry at himself for having briefly admired him.

"Oh, really? Then I suggest you go outside the hospital. There are multitudes of drug dealers who would be delighted to fill your shopping needs."

"Your other doctor helps me out."

"And who might that be?" Dean demanded. He wanted to finish up. It bothered him that this strange-looking patient was starting to negotiate with him.

Connigan began to rock back and forth in his seat mumbling to himself. A wave of pain hit Dean, nearly bending him over. He got up and hobbled to the door.

"Listen, I'll be right back. I'll look at your old chart. If what you're saying is true, we'll see. Wait here."

He staggered out, taking deep breaths. The pains subsided. He agonized whether to run to the bathroom first or to get the old chart, review it and dispose of this case. Not feeling comfortable leaving this bizarre patient alone in the exam room for any extended period of time, he decided to gamble and finish up with Connigan. Speed was definitely a priority—beads of cold sweat were beginning to pop up on his forehead.

He ran through Crawl-In, past the Big Room, ignoring the stares that followed him, and into the triage section, where the logs and old records were kept. He quickly pulled out the log book and started working his way backwards, looking for the man's name.

Ten painful minutes later he had gone two months back and not found any trace of Connigan. Frustrated, he turned to the computer, looking over records of admitted patients, clinic patients, ambulatory surgery patients. Nothing. There was no trace of the man.

Anger took over. That bum tried to scam me, he thought. It's time to kick his butt out of here.

As he turned to leave the small area, a massive cramp overtook him. Despite all self-control, a small amount of diarrhea leaked out, and for the first time since he was a young boy, Dean soiled his pants.

He went white with shame and horror. Carefully and quickly he ran out of the area, past friends and acquaintances in the Big Room who waved curious hellos, past his own section and into the linen room. There he grabbed some surgical scrubs, and he ran into the magic bathroom.

chapter 12

When he returned to his cubicle he was furious at himself and at his situation. This is not what I went to medical school for, he thought. Maybe it's time to leave this place and become a regular doctor. What's wrong with treating sore throats and blood pressure. Someone's got to do it. I've done my share of good deeds. I've helped enough poor people. Now it's time to help myself.

Angrily, he swung the door open.

"Listen, there's no record of ..."

He looked around. The room was empty. Only the odor lingered, proving that this had not been a bad dream. Otherwise, there was no trace of Connigan.

Cursing, Dean picked up Connigan's ER chart, boiling with rage. I shit in my pants for you, you dirty bastard, he thought. Uncontrollably, he threw the chart with all his might against the opposite wall. It seemed to explode on impact, papers bursting into the air. He stared at the noise, embarrassed.

He hurried over to the wall to retrieve the papers, worried that someone had heard him. I wonder what that guy was all about, he thought. He did seem to be in pain. It's probably a shame that he left. I could have done something for him. I can't believe I lost it.

As he was scooping up the last paper, he saw a small book, lying under his desk. He walked over and picked it up. Connigan had been holding a book, he thought with a frown.

It was small and badly worn, leather-bound, with loose-leaf pages. Although soiled, something about it looked like it had been lovingly used. It felt warm, soft and thick, very pleasing overall. On the front cover, carved into the leather, were engraved words. Dean squinted.

The Words of Doctor X, the title read.

What the hell is this, Dean thought. Actually, it sounds sort of interesting. Let's take a look, I'm in the mood for a good read, and I'm not going anywhere until my stomach calms down. Clinic is officially over.

He sat down and opened the book.

The first page had written on it only these words: *"Life is like Jupiter. It's a roller coaster ride through purple infinity."*

Well, thought Dean, this is indeed the professor's book. Let us proceed. He turned to the second page. On it was one line.

> *In the end the Earth will fight back. You do know that, don't you?*

Give me a break, thought Dean. Uneasily, he looked at the writing, squinting with curiosity. There was something funny about the maroon colored ink, something strangely familiar.

Suddenly he froze in disbelief. It can't be, he thought, it just can't. Instinctively, he reached into his lab coat and removed a small card and a bottle of solution. He ripped off a tiny piece of the page and put it on the card, applied a drop to it. He watched in fascination as the card turned a confirmatory blue—the words on the next few pages had been written in blood.

Dean turned the page and began to read.

> *At a crossroads we are. Midnight is either the day's end, or its beginning, and we straddle it. On Mother Nature's breaking back we have ridden to the last chapter . Full of greed, empty of vision, except maybe to rape another planet. Moon malls, can't you see it? Eve looks down on her lost paradise and cries tears of acid rain.*

*In a few years, it would anyway. Little can be done. Bear
the choking smoke, the cancerous water, with politically correct
outrage. Park by some dead river and commemorate the past. In
a few years it would end anyway.*

*May I suggest a rescue? By torchlight. Blue is the color of my
apocalyptic vision. Spot the stream with avenging warriors and
let them voyage to every corner of our gasping planet. A salvation
parented by Science and Nature, with yours truly the humble
matchmaker. Spell the Final Crusade in the sky and upon the
rich moist earth. We'll save the world. Weave your version of
what we do, be it heroism or treachery, it's all the same to me.*

*So, it begins. The madness, the shopping center/shantytown
madness will end. World, get back on your mark. Can you
remember the good old days?*

*Start the Final Crusade, then. To the soul of the jungle, I
dedicate the killing and destruction. Play once again, spirits of
the wind, and journey through your reconquered lands!*

Dean read the words over and over again, scowling. What is this?
What "Final Crusade"?

He flipped through the pages. Many were smeared with dirt or
grease. Many were filled with seemingly incoherent phrases or streams
of thought, but some were disturbingly clear.

Part of the book flowed with wild fantasies, violent or erotic. In one
passage, Connigan graphically wrote of having sex with an animal.

Another section read,

*I don't belong here. Why do I sleep in alleys, picking my
meals out of garbage cans? One thing I promise; I will escape.*

*My favorite place is always warm, and the foliage is thick
and green. The leaves are so huge you can wrap yourself up in
them. I use them when I sleep outdoors. There's no such thing as
being homeless; even the concept is humorous. . Everything is at
peace now—soon, very soon, my utopia and the earth will unite
and be one.*

Dean kept reading. He had to remind himself that he was sitting in a hospital emergency room, because he felt as if he had been swept away to another world. He was amazed at Connigan's level of alienation.

The Final Crusade of Doctor X
God created the world and loved it dearly. He bestowed upon it the gifts of color, energy and time. He let them dance to the music of the vast cosmos, and thus life was created. Nowhere else, in all the dark, endless heavens, did this happen—all else was cold hardness hurtling through eternity, obeying only the harsh, infinite laws of perfect science.

Earth. Here alone was beauty. Existence, all that ever was, all that ever mattered, was here, wildly spectacular. Every conceivable shape and color was here, and it was alive. All else was pure nothingness.

Our world sailed through time, across the blackness, with stunning, spontaneous, grace and beauty. It's impossible to grasp, in the midst of this paradise, how magnificent it all really is. Maybe it's impossible for anyone or anything to fully appreciate God's treasure. Maybe that's why we're destroying it with such ease.

Look around you. Feel the rot, smell the disintegration. It's impossible to quantify what's already been wiped out, often for reasons so trivial that it brings tears to one's eyes. We have turned our planet into a smoking ruin, and brought it to impending death. We have poisoned its land, water and air. What isn't burning up or melting is literally choking to death.

Humankind, sadly, has turned out to be an aberration, a mutation, a parasite that is rapidly strangling Earth. Despite all the evidence, which mounts daily, it continues on its nightmarish path. Within decades, if not years, the two billion year saga of our planet will be over.

We pledge ourselves to the Final Crusade. Reform is not possible. Our species is too comfort-oriented to make any real sacrifices, and it is certainly too short-sighted. The only way, the only answer, is the destruction of civilization.

The passage ended. Dean read it over and over again, trying without success to laugh at the words. Strange stuff, he thought, too strange to believe.

He flipped through the pages, ignoring the distant rumblings in his stomach. He noticed scattered lists, mostly of various chemicals and laboratory supplies, scientific calculations, and what seemed to be biochemical experiments. This stuff looks much too real for my liking, he thought uneasily.

His eyes caught on another section, one entitled, "Poisons."

> *The key is an effective, rapidly spreading virus or toxin, one easily transmitted, preferably by both air and water. Whether or not it induces pain or suffering is not important—a day or a week or a month has no relevance in the scheme of things.*
>
> *The cyanide model is a dream. It shuts down the cytochrome oxidase system, causing instant cardiopulmonary arrest. Absorbed through the skin. A lovely, neat little molecule, one part each of hydrogen, carbon and nitrogen. Easily made. The problem is the amount needed, many thousands of liters, and that it would kill animals as well as humans. Doctor X says it could be considered only for high density areas. They're devoid of most animal life, anyway.*
>
> *"Botulin toxin is another alternative. The deadliest poison available, attacking the neuromuscular junction. It would be a piece of cake to tailor- make bacteria to produce it, and we only need eight or nine liters. Again, the problem is specificity: we must target only humans."*

Dean scanned the next few pages. Many described various toxins, their mechanisms of action, the amount needed, and Connigan's personal opinion of each. Dean sensed that an enormous amount of thought had gone into this work. I actually hope that he is a crazy street person, he thought. Some of these little cocktails could kill millions, literally. And it wouldn't really be all that hard.

He turned the page and saw the words *Lac Operon*, surrounded by bloody stars and underlined. Dean felt the hair on his head begin to tingle. Something here seemed disturbingly different. Connigan mentioned "lac operon" earlier, he remembered.

> *The operon is the key to all existence as we know it. Through the induction of its genes, deep in each cell's nucleus, protein is synthesized, and chains of biochemical events are set into motion—it constitutes what we call life. The important parts for us are the operon's repressor and inducer molecules, which are derived from the i gene. They migrate to strategic parts of the DNA. The repressor finds its way to the o locus—when it's fully positioned there is no protein synthesis. The inducer has the ability to lift if off, and molecular production can resume. Block the inducer and you block activity. In other words, you block life. Everything shuts down.*

Dean shook his head, upset and frowning. This was Jacob and Monod's theory, the stuff of advanced bacterial biogenetics, and he himself understood only its rudiments. It bothered him that Connigan, a man he had practically dismissed as a ragged non-entity, could be so in command of this material. Poison descriptions could pretty much be gleaned out of any book, but this, he thought, this was pure science.

The next two lines took his breath away.

> *I have created a similar protein that binds to a parallel human repressor molecule, thus rendering it impervious, invisible, to the inducer. In short, I have discovered the antidote to human life.*

Dean couldn't stop the lump from rising in his throat.

> *My protein is human-specific. No other species are affected. I chose a remote RNA virus to produce it. I discovered it in graduate school and spent four years secretly mapping it out. No one else even knows of its existence. There's more than enough*

lead time to keep anyone from figuring it out and interfering.
My virus is both air and water borne, and can even live in the
belly of an insect. Spread from animal to person, or insect to
person, or person to person, it has a beautifully long, silent,
incubation period—completely asymptomatic victims pass it
along for days at a time. In short, it is unstoppable.

The virus has a lethality of eighty-per-cent, which is perfect.
Amongst the survivors there should be enormous secondary
mortality within a month, as the very young, the very old, and
those who need daily medications die out. At least another half
will starve. That should revert the Earth's population to Pale-
olithic levels within three months' time. We shall achieve
complete, worldwide success effortlessly. Since two picograms
are all we need per person, we need only one liter of viral
material. It's that easy. For Doctor X, I will launch a thousand
ships into the night, each filled with angels of death. And but a
few shall live …

Dean closed the book. He felt he just been on a trip to some strange
land and that he had just returned home. He wasn't sure what to do
with Connigan's writings—they were either very delusional or very dangerous, or both. There was no doubt about going to the police. The
only question was when. Although there was a contingent of hospital
security guards working now, there was only one real policeman on
patrol at night, and he was in the lobby, as was customary.

He decided to hold onto the book and return later in the morning,
when the security office would be open. He'd hand it over to Lieutenant
Brandt, who was assigned to hospital liaison matters. Let them deal
with this nonsense, he thought, I have enough trouble in my life already.

He browsed through the pages one more time. The 'end of the
world', indeed, he thought. Still, it's a provocative concept, to say the
least. What would it really be like to go back to prehistoric times. There
would be a lot more animals, I guess, but not just the cute furry ones. I
remember that picnic my ex and I took in Florida, when we set the

blanket down next to a copperhead. The world's quickest lunch. No, going back to the jungle may sound romantic and rugged, but I think I'll pass this time. Professor, I hope you really are living in a dream because you're just a little too smart for my liking.

Collecting his papers and equipment, he walked out of his cubicle and formally closed Express Care. He was now officially out sick and could do as he pleased. Because he never abused sick call he felt supremely calm and guilt-free, almost as if he were on vacation. A spasm of cramps angrily reminded him of his recent misery. Don't get too complacent, he warned himself, making a quick note of the nearest bathrooms as he walked into the Big Room and sat down in the work station.

chapter 13

As usual, there was near chaos on the air. A cardiac arrest was going on in bed six, and the area was brimming with personnel. Dean figured the patient was close to, if not already, dead, judging by the medical students jockeying around the bed with various equipment, waiting for the chance to practice some techniques on a warm body. Boy, that brings back memories. Dean thought, reminiscing about his early days. Hey, you've got to learn somewhere, and it sure beats practicing on live people.

In the adjacent beds was the usual variety of patients, known to the staff by their illnesses, such as "the pneumonia," "the gall bladder," "the shoulder," etc. It was a typical early morning.

Dean massaged his belly and to his delight the newest cramp vanished. He triumphantly waved at Finkel, who had just emerged from the arrest, pulling off his gloves. The medical students seemed to descend on the body like vampires on a fallen corpse. Finkel paid them no mind and closed the curtain. He walked over, and shook his head when he saw his friend.

"What's with you," he said. "You look like shit."

"I feel like shit."

"You going home?"

"Yeah, I can't work like this," Dean said. He hesitated for a moment. "Listen, I've got to ask you something. What would you do if you uncovered a plot to destroy mankind in order to save the rain forest?"

Finkel thought for a moment.

"I'd probably sign up with them. This world is really starting to suck."

"I'm serious."

"So am I. Do you know how long it's been since I've been laid?"

"Fink, I'm serious."

"Dean, at five a.m. nothing is serious. Okay, okay, it's a joke. Give me the punch line."

"Something really strange just happened to me. I may have uncovered some conspiracy or something."

"You've been eating jalapenos again, haven't you?"

"Just answer my question. What would you do?"

Finkel puckered his lips and thought for a second.

"Destroy the world? Maybe I'd still give the thumbs up, I don't know. Even factoring out my sex life, maybe it is time to cull the herd. Of course I don't have much friends or family, nobody likes me, and in general my life is shallow and meaningless, otherwise it might be different … Dean, what's going on?"

Briefly, Dean told his friend everything. When he was done, Finkel whistled softly and nodded his head.

"That's a good one, I'll give that to you. That tops Euler's case two months ago—you know, he had some master chef who fantasized about having sex with the food at work. I haven't been to a French restaurant since."

"Was it true?" Dean asked.

"Who knows. He told the cops. They just laughed. They probably don't eat out all that much."

"This is of far greater magnitude, you realize that, right? If this guy is for real then we're talking mass destruction."

"Well, he won't go too far without his cookbook," Finkel said. "But really, think about it. You just described a paranoid schizophrenic with an education. Big deal. A lot of them don't decompensate until well after college. It's a stretch seeing this guy in some lab mixing test tubes right now, don't you think? Relax, good buddy. You're tired, you're sick, and you just let your imagination run away from you."

Helen walked by, holding a few test tubes of blood. She noticed Dean and frowned.

"Are you okay?" she asked.

"Physically, sort of. Mentally, well, sort of."

"What are you talking about?" she asked.

Helen wore no makeup and her face was slightly lined from fatigue. But her large eyes sparkled and absently, she licked her lips. Dean had always been attracted to her, and in his exhausted state he couldn't help himself—he stared at her, entranced, desire uncomfortably tightening his chest. Whether Finkel recognized his friend's feelings or not, or whether he mistook the deep silence for mere fatigue, he awkwardly cleared his throat.

"Dean, do you mine if I tell her about the plot?" he asked Dean.

"What plot?" she asked, cocking her head.

"You've heard of the haves and the have-nots, right? Well, forget about them. The have-nothings are now on the warpath, and they're taking over the world. In fact, that overdose over there, on bed eight? He might be the commander."

Finkel then told Helen about the book. When he was done she looked at Dean, who had just doubled up with a cramp. With concern in her eyes, she reached over and gently wiped away a few beads of sweat from his forehead.

"Poor baby," she said.

"The guy may be crazy, but he's smart crazy." Dean said softly through clenched teeth. "He's not your typical street person. He uses real words. He knows his stuff. He knows all about the lac operon theory …"

"Which, if I recall correctly, does not pertain to mammalian species," Finkel interjected. "Dean, these things are a dime a dozen. A lot of people are on a conspiracy kick. We get people like this all the time."

"But usually these people feel there's a conspiracy against them," Dean argued. "This is the other way around. This man is after the whole world. Well, not the world, maybe, but most of the people in it."

"Oh, well, that makes all the difference," Finkel quipped.

"Patients with command hallucinations are potentially very dangerous," Helen agreed. "Dean, can we see the book?"

"It's hopelessly packed away," Dean said, patting his backpack as it lay on the desk. Around them swirled all types of emergencies, and Finkel started fidgeting, preparing to go out and do battle. "Anyway, whether or not it's on the level, first thing in the morning, when I wake up, I'm giving it the police."

"You do that, I'm sure they'll be duly impressed," Finkel said laconically.

"Something tells me you are not scared by all of this," Dean said, actually pleased at Finkel's unimpressed response.

"You must admit, Dean, it is a little far-fetched. You're tired, we're tired, and everything always seems worse than it is, especially in the dead of night. Frankly, I don't think things are quite as bleak as you think. This Connigan may be intelligent. But I doubt he even knows how to brush his teeth anymore."

"You think I got a little paranoid, huh?" Dean asked, smiling lightly. His friend didn't answer—Finkel was frowning at a patient on stretcher.

"Damn, look at him. You know, I was writing up his discharge when you walked by," Finkel murmured, clearly distracted. He had been watching a middle-aged man suddenly vomit, gushing dark blood onto the floor. "Talk about luck, he still has his IV. Ah yes, the Finkmaster dodges another bullet. This guy would have died at the bus stop. Thank you, Dean, for once again keeping me out of jail."

The doctor stood up and stretched his tall, lanky frame. He began to edge away from the conversation.

Dean looked at his friend. He's right, he thought. Maybe I am getting a little frazzled. Maybe deep down I'm angry at everything, and this plot or whatever it is just feeds into it.

"I see your point," he said to Finkel. The two of them walked over to the man, who was ghostly pale. Finkel examined him and wrote some orders into a chart, which he passed to Julie Shea. Dean waited patiently, and then said, "You know, Bob, it may be time for me to take that vacation, you know what I mean?"

"Absolutely," Finkel said, reaching for some chewing gum. "Hold on. Julie, tell the blood bank I want some O-negative stat, I don't want them dicking around. And send someone to Pharmacy for octreotide now. Anyway, Dean, let me say this—the professor, or whatever he is, makes some interesting points. There are too many people, and there are not enough lions, tigers and bears. Darwin never factored in all this technology and advanced medical crap. The two of us are actually a big part of the dilemma. I mean, honestly, how many people in this room should really be cured, turned loose on the street, and be allowed to reproduce? All this professor has to do is kill some doctors and the rest of the problem goes away."

"You don't have the right to make judgments like that, so don't," Helen said coolly, from several feet away from in the work station. She had been listening intently. "It's your job to keep people alive."

"I was wondering what it was," Finkel replied frostily.

"Then why do you practice medicine," Helen shot back.

Finkel glared at her. "Because it seems to me that all the saints and saviors positions are already taken, resident."

Dean stepped between them, well aware that it was fatigue causing friends' tempers to fray so badly. "Okay, okay, time out. This is just a stupid book written by a crazy person, and it's not worth any of this. I'll give it to the cops in the morning and they can figure it out."

"Good, get it over and done with," Finkel said, trying to cool off. "And now, if you'll excuse me. I'm going to save the assistant commander over there in bed two. It looks like he slashed his wrists in twenty places. He must be upset about global warming, right, Helen? Or is it what we did to the Indians?"

Helen eyed him coldly. Without a word she turned and walked away, disappearing into a cubicle. Dean could hear her well-practiced introduction to the patient inside, in a familiar singsong cadence that always seemed condescending to everyone except the patients. Suddenly a nearly instinctual alarm went off and he immediately patted his lab coat pocket—damn, damn, damn, I left my stethoscope in the exam room, he thought. Without a word he spun around and left the Big Room.

Dean rushed back to Crawl-In where he entered his cubicle and collected his piece of equipment. He thought of the book he had found. Writings of a madman, he thought to himself, half-amused. Where do people get these ideas? Someone who has trouble washing his face devises a scheme to destroy the world. Unbelievable, and in the end, very sad. Mental illness is the worst disease of them all.

As he turned around to leave, two things caught his attention. The first was that Connigan's smell was unmistakably stronger now. As if ... as if he had returned to the room while Dean was away. To get his book, he wondered, thankful for having avoided such a confrontation.

The second was a small drop of blood on his desk. He knew it was fresh because it glistened with moisture.

It hasn't even had time to clot, dean thought.

He heard a scratching sound just outside his closed door. His skin began to tingle. It suddenly occurred to him that he was alone in this remote, now closed part of the department, in the very dead of the night. For the first time in all his years here, he began to feel afraid.

Time to get out of here, he ordered himself. Swinging the door wide open, as if in denial of his mounting fear, he jumped back in shock. Standing before him was Mr. Natural. The giant guard smiled down at him.

"Sorry, Doc, didn't mean to scare you," he said, a strange look in his eyes.

"You didn't," Dean said nervously. He sensed that the other man knew otherwise.

"That guy was pretty crazy, wasn't he?"

"I guess he was a little eccentric. You said he was your friend?"

"Well, not really my friend. I knew him from the unemployment line. We had the same weekly check-in time. It became, you know, sort of like a ritual, us getting together on line and then going for a cup of coffee afterward. Yeah, eccentric, that's a good way to put it."

"Yes. Now, if you will excuse me ..."

"You don't look so good. Did that guy say anything to you? What happened?"

"I feel fine, thanks. Excuse me, but my shift is over now."

With an effort he squeezed past the giant guard, who made only the slightest of movements to let him pass through. As Dean brushed by him he caught the unmistakable odor of Connigan. Quickly, he moved away and down the hall, back to the Big Room.

"Take care, Doc, and have a nice day," he heard Mr. Natural call out behind him. "When you go to sleep, dream of beautiful things. You hear me?"

chapter 14

Dean hurried back into the Big Room, grateful for the familiar, bustling chaos all around him. Who could imagine I'd feel safe and secure in the middle of this place, he thought.

Deciding against speaking with anyone, he continued walking. As he walked down the main hallway he passed the office of his chief, Tannenbaum. He paused, making rapid mental calculations. Then he pulled a credit card from his wallet and inserted it in the door jam, snapping the lock open. He walked into the dark office and locked the door behind him.

Breaking into Tannenbaum's office was something all ER physicians were allowed to do. The chief never said quite as much, but it was a tradition. There was a wealth of textbooks in there, and it was fairly common to come in to research a difficult case or review a complex procedure before attempting it. This time, however, Dean was after something else.

He walked over to the huge copying machine and turned it on. It was known to be temperamental but now it buzzed into life. Dean sighed in gratitude. He took out Connigan's book. Quickly, and with an efficiency that surprised even himself, he made a copy of every page. The machine sputtered but obeyed; Dean patted it affectionately when he was done. He stuffed the wad of freshly copied papers in his jacket pocket, put the book back in another pocket, and let himself out.

The hallway was deserted as Dean walked towards the hospital entrance. Time to go home, he thought. As he approached the front door, a major cramp hit him. He stood there, frowning. There's no way I'm going to make it home, he thought gloomily. There's only one thing to do, he thought, go to the on-call room across the street in the resident's dorm. I'll go home in the morning and wash up.

He touched the door handle and stopped. Something was bothering him. He whirled around, and found himself staring into the wide open eyes of Mr. Natural. The guard was less than ten yards away. When he saw Dean turn around, he nodded, and lifted his hand to wave goodbye. Then he turned and went back to the ER.

Dean opened the door and bolted outside.

chapter 15

After sleeping fitfully on a lumpy cot for four hours in the rarely used on-call room—it was in fact used mostly for brief trysts between various staff members—Dean trudged to the subway for the ride home. He sat by himself, eyes half-closed with exhaustion, avoided by the other commuters who saw only a disheveled, unshaven man acting strangely.

After a long, hot shower he crashed into bed. It was delicious under the covers. God, it feels better than sex, he thought. He deliberately let himself stay awake for a few extra minutes, loving the sensation of being seduced by deep sleep. And then he let go.

At first there were no dreams. After a long while, when his tired muscles finally softened, they poured in. He found himself drifting over vast blankets of lazy steam. Everything was warm and slow moving. He swooped down and gently landed on a forest bed, and found himself amidst strange furry creatures who went quietly chewing giant green leaves. They smiled at him. He smiled back, as if he'd been here before.

One animal stopped eating and looked directly at him.

"Come on, join us. It's easier here," it whispered. "Let go."

"What are you talking about ," Dean asked.

"Connigan's right, you know, it's not worth saving," it repeated. "You tried it, it didn't work. He's not crazy, everyone else is. Don't stop him, Dean, join the Final Crusade."

"Give me one good reason," Dean said defensively. "I've got it great right where I am."

"We could give you billions." They stared at him, their glowing blue eyes piercing into him. Dean became frightened—something about them was deeply unsettling. He jumped up and starting shooting into space, flying wildly through purple void …

His telephone rang loudly, violently startling him into a sitting position. For a brief, unsettling moment he did not know where he was. Then, embarrassed at his momentary confusion, he grabbed for the phone.

"Yeah, hello?" he said, rubbing his eyes.

"Dr. Miller? Dean?" the voice said.

"Speaking."

"You sound funny. It's Dr. Tannenbaum's office."

"Hi, what's up?"

"It's five in the afternoon and you're late for your shift. It's not like you. Are you okay? They said you were sick last night."

Dean glanced at the clock on his dresser and winced. He had badly overslept. He cursed himself for not having set his alarm.

"I'll be right in," he promised.

"Thanks, the chief was getting grumpy. Normally it wouldn't be so bad, but someone else called in ~~sick~~ *late* and they're going crazy in the Big Room."

"Who called in?"

"Dr. Carpenter."

He felt a totally irrational pang of jealousy. His recent departure notwithstanding, calling in sick usually meant personal business. Rumors always seemed to swirl around Helen and her personal life. Whenever he heard any type of story about her he felt a slight bit of hurt, sometimes mixed with arousal. Dean knew how childish it was, her life was absolutely none of his business, but he couldn't help it. The gossip could easily have been false, most ER gossip was, but he still felt the mild pain every time he listened.

"I'm on my way," he said flatly.

He sat in the middle of the bed, not wanting to move. How about something to eat on the way to work, he mused. What does one eat at this hour after sleeping the day away, breakfast or dinner?

After shaving he walked over to the closet and reached blindly for a shirt. To his surprise he pulled out a pair of pants. He stared at them. No way, he thought. I'm not the world's neatest guy, but I keep them on the right side and this is the left.

He reached for another hanger, and the same thing happened. What the hell, he wondered, and he swung the closet door wide open.

His clothes had been completely reversed. What's going on, Dean thought uneasily. I've used this system for months, years.

He dressed quickly, staring continually at his clothes, as if they could somehow give him an answer. He looked at his apartment. Nothing seemed out of place. On an impulse he walked over to his desk. It seemed to be in order. He opened a drawer, the one containing papers, in which normally were carelessly tossed inside. They were now neatly stacked and arranged.

He scanned the apartment, almost expecting to be rushed. The room was very still. Dean stared at his bed, at the blankets draped over it, tumbling onto the floor. He was terrified at the thought of lifting them and looking underneath. His eyes wide with fear and confusion, he grabbed his backpack and hurried out.

chapter 16

Jack, the newly christened Death Master, waited patiently by the elevator, groaning under the weight of his grocery bags. He leaned against the wall-length mirror, feeling slightly uncomfortable in the apartment building's well-appointed lobby. He stared at the floor numbers changing on the electronic wall button, trying to will the elevator down. Next to him were two men, back from a hard day's work. They obviously didn't know each other, but they kept together, clearly shunning this apparent delivery man. Jack could feel hatred for them welling up inside, leaving a bitter taste in his throat.

He stole a few glances at them. Both were tall, taller than him, in their late twenties, well dressed and well built. Yuppie muscles, he thought scornfully. Good for nothing but looking good.

The two men seemed to exude success. One was deeply tanned and very handsome, with thick black hair, carefully slicked back. He was wearing expensive jewelry and wore a flowing camel hair coat that made Jack feel ashamed in his army field jacket. The other man had thinning red hair, tortoise shell glasses and a neatly trimmed beard. A wise ass, Jack thought. I bet this guy thinks he's real smart.

The three moved towards the door when the elevator arrived. The two businessmen politely stepped aside to let this delivery man enter first. With a grunt he obliged, trying to control his anger. Keep cool, the hunter said to himself, this is business. The two men quietly followed, lost in thought. The door closed and the elevator began to ascend.

Instantly Jack dropped his bags. He pushed the stop button and in the same movement punched the black-haired man squarely in the face. His fist made a cracking sound as it hit the point of the nose. The seasoned fighter had aimed it right—his victim crashed back in shock and pain, and then crumpled to the floor. The other man froze with horror, unable to even lift his hands. Jack turned to him and whipped a left hook into his temple. The red haired man collapsed, half with fear, half with pain.

"Give me your wallet now!" Jack shouted. "Now!"

The man, pale with terror, clumsily fumbled for his breast pocket. Jack pushed his trembling hand away and ripped out his wallet. He then reached for the man's watch. Instinctively, the man pulled back his wrist. Enraged, Jack reached into his grocery bag and pulled out a large can. He started beating the man, smashing it into the wailing man's head again and again. Finally, the man stopped crying and lay still.

The Death Master knelt down and removed the watch, then turned to the other man, who was still unconscious. He quickly searched him, removing anything of value. Finally, he turned to the man's huge gold ring, studded with diamonds. His eyes gleamed. I want that ring, he thought, grabbing it. But tugging and pulling were to no avail. Whipping out a pair of wire cutters, he lined them up against the man's finger. He squeezed with all his might.

A dull crunching sound filled the elevator cabin as the blade went through the bone. In a moment the finger fell to the ground, the ring still on it. Jack plucked the finger off the floor and put it in his pocket.

He pushed the stop button back and the elevator began to move. His last action was to very carefully remove the man's camel haired coat. To his delight no blood had gotten on it. What made him even happier was that there was no one on the fourteenth floor when the elevator stopped. This was always the great unknown in operations like these— you could find yourself in staring into a group of ten people or into the face of a cop. He pushed each floor button to insure the longest ride for his victims, grabbed a bag of groceries and walked outside. The door closed behind him.

Looking down the hallway, he saw a woman wearing only pajamas taking a bag of garbage to the incinerator room. She looked at him quizzically. He looked at her, considering whether or not he should rush her and drag her into her apartment for some fun. But he had to hurry— police would no doubt be here in fifteen minutes. What a shame, he thought, I'm in the mood for love ...

"Excuse me, ma'am? Is this the fifteenth floor?" he asked politely.

"No, no it's not," she answered, relieved at his civility. She smiled at him. "We're on fourteen."

"Oh my goodness, I've done it again. Guess I'll walk up," he said lightly. "Gotta walk off this fat. The only exercise I get lately is lifting potato chips into my mouth."

The woman laughed."Now, now, you've got to have will power."

"You know, you're right. Have a nice day ma'am. Sorry to bother you."

"You take care," she said graciously.

He quickly entered the stairway, dropping his bag, and scrambled down, taking three or four steps at a time. In a minute he was back at the lobby. Calmly, he walked out of the building. The doorman didn't even look up from his paper as he passed by.

In the street Jack breathed deeply, letting the cool twilight air chill and tingle his skin. He indulged himself for a few seconds in front of the building, reviewing in his mind the highlights of this fresh victory, daring anyone to capture him. And then he strode off towards his car, the one he had stolen earlier that day.

He was exhilarated from his triumph. The master has done it again, he exulted, fondling the camel hair coat. It took effort to not skip down the street.

Rounding the corner he grinned broadly when he noticed that his car still had twenty minutes left on the parking meter. I'm so law abid- ing I can't stand it, he snickered. And now for a soothing drive out of here.

He opened the door and slid in. After stretching lazily he reached into his pocket and pulled out the finger. Quickly he extracted the ring, putting the finger in the ashtray, laughing at the thought of maybe placing it in a pack of cigarettes and using it as a practical joke. We're gonna have some fun tonight, he said to himself. Placing his left hand on the steering wheel, he reached forward with his right to hot-wire the engine.

He frowned. The steering wheel was sticky with some type of resin or glue, and his hand was covered with it. Jack stared at his hand. It felt warm and numb. Damn, he thought, this shit is weird.

Rubbing his palm on his pants didn't help; the resin practically seemed to melt into his skin. His hand suddenly fell to his side, unable to move, and to his horror a burning sensation began creeping up his arm. Get out of the car, get out of the car, he said to himself, but to his horror his arm had gone dead and he couldn't open the door. He whispered out loud, "What is going on, what in God's name is going on?"

The paralyzing fire reached his shoulder and paused for a moment. Then it erupted, branching out into his neck and chest. All the man could do was sit in frozen disbelief as his body became limp, and he crumpled forward, fully alert, into the steering wheel.

Within seconds the paralysis was complete. Jack lay still, focusing all his thoughts on his struggle to breathe. His lips couldn't move, but his mind was screaming in absolute, uncontrollable terror. When he sensed his car door flying open, and his helpless body being dragged from the car, he could do nothing to protect himself. He felt himself beginning to suffocate and barely noticed when he was thrown in back of what seemed to be a truck. His last sensations before he lost consciousness were that of a breathing mask held tightly over his face, forcing air into his mouth and nose, and bouncing up and down as the truck raced down the street.

chapter 17

To Dean's great annoyance, his train stopped between stations, making what was normally a quick relatively pleasant trip seem like a long marathon. Dean fumed. He was already late, and this was developing into his worst case scenario. With maximum effort he forced himself to calm down. Once upon a time, he thought, you walked out of your house, or your hut, or cave, or whatever, and you were there. This commuting is for the birds.

He hated the subway. This particular car was relatively clean, and there were only a few possibly dangerous people on it. Several feet away from him a raggedly-dressed man slept, sprawled out over several seats. Dean was positive he had recently treated this person for an overdose, and prayed that the man would not wake up and recognize him.

As was his habit, he started fantasizing about his dreams from the night before. He half closed his eyes, part of him monitoring the potential threats all around him, the rest of him locked deep in his faraway world, where he had no fears or insecurities. When his train finally crept into his station, he got up with a tinge of sadness and walked out.

After rushing from the station to the hospital, Dean stopped at the security office, panting. With dismay he realized that it was closed for the day. What a drag, he thought. Not only am I late, but I'm stuck with Connigan's book for another day.

Mumbling angrily to himself, he pulled an apple from his pack and headed for the linen room to get a white coat—this was the only dress requirement of the department. Often, it was all that distinguished some doctors, like Finkel, from their patients.

Surprisingly, Tannenbaum was standing there, as if waiting for him. Dean was astounded—he had never seen his chief anywhere but in his office or at departmental meetings, except for occasional forays into the ER itself. More than that, this was after regular hours. Dean was used to working irregular hours—for many years he had worked half of all weekends and holidays, and almost that many nights. But no one minded that Tannenbaum did not work them, or for that matter, even see patients anymore—he had paid his dues in the trenches, all agreed, and he had made it easier for all who followed him—*he* was entitled to a "day job."

The older man extended his hand, and the two hands shook awkwardly. Dean had found the ER director a painfully shy man, not aloof or imperious as others thought. Unless there was business to discuss it was always difficult talking to him, there being such a stiff, cardboard quality to every encounter.

"Dean, how are you?" Tannenbaum asked.

"Hanging in there."

"Is everything going all right for you in the ED?" his chief asked, using the more appropriate abbreviation, standing for emergency department, "Are there any issues?"

"I guess everything is pretty much the same."

One had to be on full alert when discussing matters with Tannenbaum. It was forbidden to make jokes or pass judgment about any patient. One doctor recently had been severely reprimanded for calling one a bum. "We're not God," the chief would sternly lecture, "We're not here to judge, that will happen the day they die. We're physicians, we exist only to treat the patient."

The more radical doctors fully endorsed this position, and the rest, whose middle class values were usually tested to their limit in this inner city world, had learned to live with it. In this ER, doctors typically looked around them before joking about a patient, in much the same way racial remarks commonly began elsewhere. As Finkel was fond of saying, keep what you say short, to the point, and politically correct.

After the slightest of pauses Tannenbaum cleared his throat.

"Dean, did you treat a patient named John Connigan last night?"

Dean was surprised—his chief rarely, if ever, seemed aware of the details of his department, being nearly consumed with meetings, turf battles with other departments, interviews and policy matters. The question immediately put him on guard.

"Yeah, I saw him for a headache," he answered carefully, knowing it was useless to lie about such an obvious fact.

"Did you have any problem with him?"

"He eloped on me, just walked out. Does that count as a problem?"

"Did he say anything?"

"He said quite a few things. Why are you asking?"

"He's dangerous, Dean, delusional, with paranoid tendencies. He also has a doctorate in virogenentics."

"I know that."

"You do? Dean, there have been rumors that this man is planning to dump something, some poison, in a reservoir. If he said anything pertinent to that last night, if is there any information you can give …"

"This may be for real?" Dean asked. He felt partly relieved that his concern about Connigan had been legitimate after all. He also felt a pang of anxiety when he thought of his apartment, of it having been possibly broken into. The book suddenly felt heavier in his pocket. Get rid of it, he thought.

"Listen, maybe they can use this. I think Connigan dropped it on his way out last night."

He pulled the book out and handed it over to his chief, who stared intently at the pages. His eyes seemed to bulge slightly as he perused it.

"It's just a lot of mumbo jumbo, but maybe they can make some sense out of it," Dean said. "I know I couldn't."

Tannenbaum flipped through the pages, nodding his head.

"The ravings of a lunatic," he murmured.

Dean was shocked at the word. Connigan must be a special case indeed, he thought.

"There's nothing really conclusive in the writings, but it does show intent," Dean said, trying to be helpful. "No one believed me last night."

"You read this … did you show it to other people?"

"Well, yeah, why not. It seemed like a big joke."

"If it's all right with you, I want to call Officer Brandt at home and arrange to give him this book. Time may be a factor here."

"Sure, I was actually coming in to give it to him. I guess I'm a little late. Sorry about that, by the way."

"Don't worry, it happens to everyone. I assume you will be available if there are any further questions?"

"I don't think it would do any good. I don't know anything else."

"Of course." Tannenbaum shuffled subtly, indicating that the conversation was ending. "This is all silly junk, Dean, we see this once in a while. Insanity, isn't it, this ending the world stuff."

"Maybe, but I'm sure some people out there think the world would be a lot better off without us. For them, species suicide might be a true philosophical question. Connigan might be one of them"

"Dean, if you can, drop this matter. It's pointless stirring things up. The department does not need this publicity, within the hospital or the community. Anyway, it was good speaking with you. If anything does develop regarding this, which I doubt, I'll keep you informed."

Tannenbaum turned around and disappeared down the hall. Dean stood there, wondering if he had done the right thing. How does he know about Connigan, he wondered. I know he's a committed environmentalist, but this stuff is above and beyond …

He was interrupted by a nurse's aide, who seemed to have been searching for him.

"Dr. Miller, there you are. Doctor Molloy is looking for you."

"I bet. Be right there."

Well, time to rescue people trying to kill themselves, he thought. Thank goodness for drugs, alcohol and tobacco, otherwise I'd be flipping burgers. At least this will take my mind off things. Good-bye, Doctor X, hello blood and guts.

He walked towards the ER, occasionally looking around him to make sure he wasn't being watched or followed. And then, patting the copy of Connigan's book in his pocket, he took a deep breath, opened the door into the main ER and went to work.

Dean walked into the work station, disgusted with himself. Not only was he significantly late, which was just about the worst sin an ER doctor could commit, he had done nothing since his last shift here but sleep—it was as if he had never left.

He took a tense signout from a tight-lipped colleague, Carl Molloy, who had been waiting for him. Dean could sense the doctor was trying hard not to show anger. I really can't blame him, Dean thought. You pace yourself for a marathon, and then you're asked to run a little more, when there's no more to give. He barely listened, knowing he'd be re-starting all the cases practically from scratch. When the report was complete, the tired doctor grimly shuffled away, and Dean sat down, trying to psyche himself up for another long haul.

"Miller, spend a little more time with your medicine and less with your fantasy life, okay?" Molloy asked cuttingly over his shoulder as he left.

"You're not so perfect yourself, Molloy," Dean snapped. "This isn't the end of the world, you know."

The two had never gotten along. The doctor turned back to glare at him.

"It is when I stick around this hole one minute longer than I have to!"

With that Molloy spun around and walked out angrily.

Dean slumped in his chair and looked around, taking the sights and sounds about him. He heard bits of conversations from all sides.

"… Julie, you could wear that dress."

"God, no, it's too green. Turn the page."

Another nurse said, "So I called the registrar to check on my kid, and you know what? In two years of college she's gotten only eight credits. Eight credits!"

From another angle, he heard someone say, "Of course the city was better twenty years ago. Everything was better twenty years ago."

"Dude, have a snack."

Dean turned around. Finkel approached with a bag of freshly microwaved popcorn. The smell was pure nighttime ER—he had lost all taste for it outside of work because he identified with it so strongly here. Politely he grabbed a handful. Finkel motioned with his head, and Dean turned to see a red-haired woman with a clipboard walk by, examining patients' trays.

"I want to eat the nutritionist," Finkel lustily whispered, staring at her.

Dean nodded his agreement and took another handful. It had been more than six months since his marriage had ended, and he was at the point now where he was deeply interested in every nearly woman he saw.

"So, you have any interesting cases lately," he asked, trying to change the subject.

"If I did, I missed 'em," Finkel absently replied, sitting down. He kept his eyes on the woman until she walked around a corner. Then he sighed loudly.

"Hey, it's the drug pusher Gus," he called out merrily to a nearby pharmacist, a white haired man putting various pills in the medication bin. The elderly man waved at him and smiled. "Tell the truth now, Gus, there ain't nothing like a good come, right?"

"Dear boy, when you get to be my age, you're going to find that the greatest thing in life is taking a big dump," the man replied. All three of them laughed.

"And I see you and Molloy are still as friendly as ever." Finkel mumbled through a half stuffed mouth, while they munched on the popcorn. "Ignore him, Dean, rumor has it he's interviewing downtown. I say, good riddance."

"For once, I'm actually inclined to agree with him. I can't believe I overslept."

The ER was amazingly empty, a true rarity, and Dean and Finkel finished the popcorn, languidly looking around them. Gloria, the housekeeper, slept by another desk, her head resting on folded arms. Only the unit secretary seemed alive, talking and laughing passionately over the phone. Her legs were crossed, and Dean was annoyed at his inability to keep from staring at them. It seemed as if they possessed a mysterious force which had locked onto his eyes. He felt his chest tighten with each peek, and several times he fought the urge to throw his entire career away and jump on her. With ultimate effort he willed himself to look away, feeling pained but triumphant at this remarkable self-control.

Helen walked over, and he inwardly groaned as his sexual urges once again bubbled to the surface. She looked beautiful tonight, and her lips looked softer, and her eyes more sparkling, than ever. She pulled up a chair and sat down in the style of a man, swinging her leg around the seat.

"How you feeling?" she asked.

"Better," he answered, uncertain of how to answer.

"Is all that stuff from last night taken care of?" she asked.

"Stuff? The cramps are gone. The book's done with. The police have it and just maybe I'm done with conspiracies. At least, I hope I am. Tannenbaum's in charge of the case."

"What do you mean," Helen asked quizzically.

Finkel leaned forward. "That's right, I forgot. Dean, you saved the world last night."

"Very funny. In any event, listen to this. I think someone broke into my apartment last night while I was away?"

"You were robbed?" Helen asked, squinting her eyes.

"I don't know, all they seemed to do was re-arrange things, in my closet, my desk. No one took anything. Maybe it's some sort of weird birthday present or something, you know, you read about these things sometimes. Only it's not my birthday."

"Someone re-arranged your closet," Finkel nodded. "And your desk. How nefarious. Dean, I'm starting to worry about you."

"I don't know what to say, it really happened."

"Sounds like my mother knocked off your place," Finkel continued. "She'll break under questioning. Of course, she's in Florida, this may be difficult."

"Fink, this is serious."

"Why would anyone do something like that?" Helen asked with concern.

"I don't know, but this book thing occurred to me. Maybe they were after that. Everyone in the ER heard me talk about it."

"So they sent in an Amazonian cleaning lady, is that it?" Finkel added in mock horror. "Oh, those dirty bastards, they sure know how to play rough."

"Was anything missing?" Helen asked, ignoring him.

"I don't know, I just got out of there. I was scared, and to top it off I was late …"

Suddenly the code phone rang. Finkel shot up to get it, not out of urgency or panic, but out of superstition—he absolutely had to pick up between the first and second ring.

"Central. Yeah … okay … when? … what's your ETA … thanks."

He hung up and turned to the expectant staff. Reaching into his shirt pocket he took out a stick of gum and put it in his mouth . They knew what he was going to say.

"Sixty-two year old male. Full arrest, witnessed. Showtime in four to five."

"Julie, call the code," Ehler said, walking over. He turned to Dean and whispered, "Finally, something to break up the day. You want to run it, it will get your mind off this silliness. No offense meant, really."

"None taken. Dan, I know it's weird on my part. Maybe part of me deep down wants everything to just start all over, and this book just played into that. I guess I should call it what it is, and that's depression. But anyway, thanks for the offer—with my luck the code will last an hour, and I'm behind already," Dean said. "You mind running it?"

"No, of course not. There's this great article in the *Annals* which gives a new protocol for pulseless electrical activity. We'll give it a shot. And you know, Dean, let's not call it depression. Why don't we just say you're a little burnt out right now, and leave it at that. Okay?"

Helen continued writing on her chart, Gloria remained asleep, and everyone else got up and walked into the Code Room, going to their assigned spots. Seconds later, Harry the medical student shyly entered, followed by a stern looking nurse supervisor; the doctors paid her little mind, but the nurses and the ancillary staff shifted uneasily and checked their uniforms and ID badges the moment she appeared.

Dean got up and stretched. "I'll be the welcoming committee. Helen, let's get some fresh air."

She smiled at him and put down her chart. Together they walked through the electronic doors into the warm twilight. The ambulance port faced west, in front of them was the parking lot. The darkening violet sky was rimmed with red and orange, and above them black clouds twisted silently. The air was thick and soft, the breeze that carried it sweet and palpable. A siren bubbled in the distance. They leaned against a wall, their shoulders touching ever so slightly.

"It's a shame to die on a night like this," Dean said to himself quietly.

He felt very comfortable with her and wished there was something he could do to make her attracted to him. Sometimes he could sense her actually trying to feel affection, but it was of no use. They remained good friends, albeit in the workplace, each of them not even knowing where the other lived.

"I hope whoever rolls in, he did everything he wanted to," she said.

Both knew that the chances of reviving a street arrest at best slim, and the chances of a full save, with the patient eventually walking out of the hospital intact, practically nil. With a combination of medical talent and good or bad luck, depending on one's perspective, at best this person would wind up a vegetable in the ICU.

At that moment the ambulance pulled into the parking lot, its red lights sparkling. Marking a surprisingly graceful maneuver, it turned around and glided backwards into the port. Inside they could see figures moving up and down, no doubt paramedics pumping on the patient's chest.

Although he'd worked on hundreds of arrests, Dean still felt the momentary surge of excitement which he saw the medics run around and open the doors, revealing the melodrama inside. Yup, he thought, time to duke it out with death one more time.

"Greetings and salutations," he called out as they approached, pushing the stretcher. "Welcome to our humble inn."

The medics smiled and nodded to him. Dean was one of the few doctors who treated them as true professionals, not resenting their field efforts like other doctors did, who mostly felt they should do little more than scoop and carry. Dean considered them members of the same team, and underpaid and overworked to boot. For this they were profoundly grateful.

The team rushed the stretcher past him. Dean was curious as to what had happened and decided to observe for a while. Why not, he said to himself, it's a slow night. He followed the crew into the Code Room, nodding his good-bye at Helen, who shook her head, indicating she wanted to remain outside. I might as well go inside, he thought, it hurts being around her.

"So what surprise did you bring us tonight?" he heard Ehler asking casually. "And I see that Dean had decided to give us the pleasure of his company after all. You just can't stay away from these fun and games, can you?"

Deftly, Ehler interviewed the medics on the details, such as down time, meds given en route, past medical history. Seconds later the medics left, their job done. The door closed.

After an initial surge of action, consisting of additional IV lines being placed, cardiac monitors being strapped on, and the patient being intubated, the actual resuscitation began. The basic team was there, along with a few curiosity seekers from other departments, there on the premise of asking if their services were needed—after a few minutes they trickled out, secretly satisfied.

Ehler stood by the old, squeaking EKG machine, giving medication orders. Finkel wandered in, munching on popcorn and stood next to Carol, who stayed by the crash cart, with Julie administering the medications as ordered. A respiratory technician pumped air into the patient's endotracheal tube, and the medical student, Harry, was dutifully pumping on the chest. He grunted from the exertion, beads of sweat dripping from his nose onto the patient. He secretly didn't mind this as he was on a diet and had been wracked with guilt after having just gorged on junk food.

After the nurse supervisor left, the group collectively smiled. Finkel was the first to speak. The code was proceeding without much success.

"Hey, this guy is really dead," he said. "We're not even close. Julie, darling, pull another atropine out of that magical cart."

"You got it."

"How many minutes has it been." Ehler asked.

"Twelve," Carol answered, looking at the wall clock.

"Let's go another eight."

The entire group shrugged.

"Atropine given," Julie said.

"Julie, you give good atropine."

"Oh, that's not all I give that's good, Dr. Finkel."

Everyone laughed.

The patient passed flatus loudly. And then did it once again. Every time Harry compressed his chest the man passed gas, his stomach and intestines having filled the air during the ambulance ride, from his face mask having pushed air into both the stomach and lungs. Now, every time his chest was compressed, he was expelling it.

"God, not again," Finkel muttered. He looked at the student. "Harry, this happens every time you do CPR. I think you have some kind of curse. And just when I was going to make a move on Julie. How can I be romantic with this kind of ambiance?"

Dean looked down at the man. Clean shave, he thought. Clean socks. This guy had no idea this was his final day on earth.

"Hey, you want to hear the latest disaster in Eastside's ER?" Carol asked. "This ten month old comes in with severe asthma, I heard he was practically blue. They wheel him down to X-ray after one lousy treatment and leave him in the hall, unescorted and off any monitor. Of course he stops breathing, it's at least five minutes before anyone realizes it, and it's another five before he's intubated. They couldn't find the introsseous kit, so some resident tries to start a subclavian line, gives the kid a pneumothorax, and the attending puts the chest tube in the wrong side. The wrong side!"

"A subclavian, huh. What did he use, a butterfly needle?" Finkel asked sarcastically.

" Needless to say, the kid died."

"I'm shocked and appalled." Finkel said dryly.

Harry stopped pumping for a second and looked at Carol. "Wow," he breathed.

Finkel snorted with laughter. "Inefficiency at its very best. Even I'm impressed. Let's have an epinephrine, please."

"It goes to show what kind of shop Bradley runs over there," Ehler said. "I tell you, his left ball doesn't know what his right ball is doing."

"Epinephrine given," Julie said.

"Do you realize that this man is wearing clean socks?" Dean suddenly commented. Everyone turned to him.

"Oh my goodness, are we getting heavy again?" Finkel asked with mock suffering. "Dean, must we discuss the secrets of the universe during every arrest?"

"And he shaved," Dean continued. "Not in his wildest dreams did he realize that this would be his last day. Would you change your socks if you knew you were going to die?"

"Hell, no, I'd be running around naked, boinking everybody. Right, Carol?"

"And I'd be helping you out, honey," she said, smiling.

Dean looked at Ehler. "What would you do on your last day?"

"I think Finkel has the right idea," Ehler said. "But if I know my wife, she'd spend her last day cleaning. She'd probably make me help her."

"Carol, it's your turn."

"I'd go back to smoking and eat a lot of ice cream."

The dead man farted.

They stopped talking for a moment, the only sounds in the room the squeak of the old EKG machine and rhythmic hiss of the rubber bag squeezing air into the patient's lungs.

"Dean, you've been torturing us during codes for years now," Finkel said. "So, tell us, what really is the secret of life?"

"Well, for one thing, don't die in a hospital."

"I think that's pretty much a given. Even you, Harry, you know that by now, right?" Finkel exclaimed. "That's just the bare bones, Dean, we want the meat. Come on, what is the point to all this."

An aide came in, holding a driver's license.

"We have a name on this guy," he said. "James Larsen."

Everyone looked at the patient, for a moment regarding him as a real person and not just some anonymous slab of human flesh thrown into their midst. As often happened there was a collective pang of guilt over the irreverence with which he had been treated.

He was a large, thickly built man with short white hair and a square face. Although his massive chest and arms were now soft and fat, it was apparent that once he had been a bull. I bet he was once a king of this world, Dean thought. One day, we all fall off the mountain.

He walked to the head of the stretcher and stared into the man's purplish face. He looked at the mottling of the torso, shaking his head with the barest of movements.

"I know what you're thinking," Ehler said. "This thing was over before it began.

Dean, while you're up here, check the carotids. Harry, stop your pumping."

"Splendid. Keep going, Harry. I'm going try out this new recipe."

He smiled and pulled out a folded article out of his pocket. He whispered something to Julie, who opened a drawer on the crash cart.

"By the way, Dr. Finkel, we all saw the way you were making bedroom eyes at the nutritionist," Julie said in mock jealousy, while filling a syringe.

"Wrong, Julie, they were not bedroom eyes. They were bathroom eyes."

"Dr. Ehler, what did you think of her," Julie asked mischievously.

"I'm now allowed to think of her. I'm married." the doctor murmured, filling a syringe with a clear fluid.

"You don't have to look around," Julie said. "Your wife is very cute."

"She irons underwear."

"Oh, I bet she's very sexy."

"She irons underwear."

"There's more to love than just sex, anyway," Julie said.

"Says who," Finkel asked.

"Says me," Julie stuck her jaw out defiantly, trying hard not to smile.

"Just give me one example of what is more important than sex," Finkel said.

"Well, you may think I'm old fashioned, but I don't care. I think snuggling after sex happens to be more important than the sex itself."

"And I know for a fact that post-coital snuggling happens to be unnatural," Finkel retorted.

"Why is it unnatural?" asked Julie, perplexed.

"If God meant for there to be snuggling after sex, He wouldn't have made the wet spot so cold."

"Isn't it time for another atropine?" Carol asked, rolling her eyes in exasperation.

"Here goes," Ehler said. "Four grams of magnesium, two milligrams of glucagon, going in."

"Where on earth did you read that ... hey, what's the soup today in the cafeteria?" Finkel asked, looking at his watch.

"Chicken gumbo," Harry replied.

Several people made faces.

"Again?" Finkel said incredulously. "Dean, talk about conspiracies."

Dean looked down into the man's face, slowly shaking his head.

"I'm taking a poll," he murmured, half to himself. "What do you think is the best way to die?"

Finkel and Ehler exchanged weary glances; the metaphysician was at it again. The others giggled uncomfortably. Harry stopped pumping and looked at Dean, trying to think of an answer.

"Do you accept things like 'over and under two nineteen year olds,'" Finkel asked.

"No, I want a serious answer."

"Dean, I haven't been serious for years," Finkel asked. "Excuse me, Harry, your patient needs some compressions. May we pump a little, please?"

"Anyone?" Dean asked, looking around. Harry resumed his pumping, sneaking a quick look at the wall clock.

"There's got to be a vaccine for this," Finkel whispered to Ehler.

"Well, for starters, I wouldn't want to die in a hospital, with someone pounding on my chest," Julie said, coming to Dean's aid.

"Hold it a second," Finkel said, looking at the EKG rhythm strip. Harry paused gratefully. "Nah, still dead. Pump for a few more minutes. You think we ought to pace Big Jim?"

"He's too far gone," Ehler said, shaking his head. "His down time was too long."

"All right, let's go five more."

Ehler cleared his throat.

"I'd go to a beach house somewhere in the tropics, with a good bottle of scotch and some great books …"

"Short books, I assume," interrupted Finkel. "Hey, what's this? Stop pumping. Nope, just artifact. Continue pumping. Sorry, Dan, go on with your last day on this planet."

"There isn't much more. I'd just hang out, enjoying the view. I am allowed to fade away, aren't I, or do you want an actual cause of death."

Dean turned to Julie.

"Pneumonia," she said. "Anytime after I get to kiss my great-grand-daughter."

"You're kidding," Carol said. "You want people to remember you as a two-legged prune?"

"The way I see it, I'll be dead for a very long time. I'll stay down here as long as I can, thank you. And I've never seen a happy dead person, have you?"

They stared at the patient.

"You guys ready for me?" Finkel asked, looking around.

"I don't know if I'm ready for this," Carol said. "Okay, honey, why don't you tell us."

"I want to be, oh, about sixty-eight, sixty-nine, right before you start to shrivel. I'll go to, you know Mexico, go to some brothel, a cantina, get roaring drunk, have as much sex as my aging dick will allow, and then go into the desert and die in a gun battle. You know, with all the glory, me against the bad guys. Something like the Alamo."

They stared at him.

"You want to die in a gun battle?" Carol said, looking at him with astonishment. "This is what goes on in that little brain of yours?"

"Doctor Ehler?"

"What," he replied dryly, looking at the weary student, whose glasses slipped down to the very tip of his nose.

"It's been twenty minutes."

"So it has. Stop pumping. Nothing on EKG. Check the lead placement. No, still flat."

As was Ehler's custom, he looked around the room. There was a trace of seriousness in his eyes. He was going to end the code in his customary manner and officially declare the man dead.

"Does anyone object to stopping?"

There was silence.

"Then it's over. Thank you, everyone." He tapped the body's toes. "Bon voyage, Mr. Larsen. Darn, the recipe didn't work."

"Hey, maybe you could use it to punch up a brownie mix," Finkel suggested.

The mood of the room changed instantly, as the outside world of the ER roared back into everyone's thoughts. Wordlessly, Finkel, Ehler and Harry walked out. Julie and an ER tech began to clean up the body, making faces at all the blood and excretions on the sheets. Carol continued to chart.

Helen walked into the room. She ignored the body and smiled at Dean.

"There you are. I thought you weren't going to work on the code."

"He wasn't," Carol said, not looking up from her clipboard. "He was taking confession."

"Come with me," Helen said. "I'm having trouble with a dislocated thumb."

"Yeah, sure, these sometimes need the OR," he said. He looked at the nurses. "Ta ta, everyone."

"Wait a minute, wait a minute," Julie protested. "You didn't tell us how you wanted to die."

Helen looked at him quizzically.

"I want to die saving the world," he said.

"What does that mean?" Julie asked.

Dean thought of Connigan's book. "I'm not sure yet. But I'll let you know."

"You doctors are so strange," Carol said, never taking her eyes off the chart.

Dean smiled and left the room.

chapter 18

John Connigan tapped meekly on the front door in the approved sequence, three, one, one, three. He had walked to this lonely looking house from the train station, nearly five miles away, in a steady drizzle and looked even more bedraggled than usual. His clothes were soggy and a drop of water ran down his face, smearing his glasses with muddy streaks. He had tripped several times during his long walk here, simply because he could not see anything, and there were new rips in his already tattered clothing.

Connigan shuffled nervously—it was forbidden to come to headquarters uninvited. There was an electronic click and the door opened. Tentatively he entered and closed the door behind him. There was another electronic click.

The dark hallway he stood in appeared empty. Very carefully, so as not to trip, he made his way into an adjacent room. The thick, light-proofed curtains were tightly drawn; only a dim lamp resting on a table let him see where he was. Aside from the table, there were only a few wooden folding chairs and a large soft couch. He walked over to it and with a heavy grunt, sat down.

The silence was so thick that he swore he could see and hear it, and feel it rushing through him like a river. He self-consciously sniffled, and scratched his scalp, embarrassed at the noise he made. After a few minutes he relaxed, letting the tomblike stillness envelope and take control of him as he waited in the semi-darkness.

So peaceful, he thought. Like the caves I used to run away to. I'm glad the Final Crusade will take place in a cave when it's complete, it will feel like going home. It will be so peaceful there. The devil created noise and God created images. If I could spacewalk, the first thing I'd do would be to cut the rope and fly into quiet eternity. It would be delicious, drifting through the void into nothingness. Let the universe be my resting place, the infinite cosmos my soft deathbed.

He closed his eyes, licked his lips, and found himself shooting past spinning asteroids and sparkling comets as he headed towards a cold, faraway star. So lovely, he sighed. Life is like Jupiter. A roller coaster ride through purple infinity.

"So you're back."

Connigan started. Seated in front of him was Mr. Natural, who was looking at him icily.

"Please don't hit me again."

"You're not supposed to come here."

"I want to see Doctor X."

"Doctor X doesn't want to speak to you." Mr. Natural leaned forward. "They're on to us, you know. All thanks to you."

"I'm sorry. I was in so much pain that night I didn't know what I was doing."

"You may have blown everything. And I'm in hot water for having steered you to that do-gooder Miller."

"Then you shouldn't have brought me to him."

"I never thought you'd give him the fucking book!" the guard snapped.

"I'm so sorry. You have no idea how I feel."

"I couldn't care less how you feel. We have to rush now. No more human models after the ones downstairs—the risk is now too high. Thanks to you. We'll release some virus on the streets and see if we can brew some mini-epidemic or something. That's the best we can do now. We'll observe the results from the field. So much for any scientific projections regarding infectability, mean lethal dose and all that other crap you keep talking about.

"Actually, in a day or two we were coming to get you," Mr. Natural continued, in a business-like manner. "As of now you're grounded. You are to stay here until we successfully incorporate the histidine complex into the viral RNA."

"That could take forever," Connigan protested nervously. "The process only seems to work at a pH greater than 7.50. I need more time to ..."

"You don't have any more time," Mr. Natural growled. "You spent the last of it in that emergency room. We figure on two weeks at the most before we're discovered. You will, I repeat, you will make it work, and in the very near future."

Mr. Natural's voice softened.

"John, listen. Some very intelligent people have come across your writings. You put everything in that book, from the overall scope of the plan down to the coded time and place of release. You put it all in there, you told me that in the ER room, remember? Is this address also in that book?"

"I don't think so."

"Whatever. One of the labs or supply houses will point the way if nothing else does. There's just no time any more. We've got to get out of here. And if anyone comes looking for us, I'll just have to take care of them."

"Don't hurt anyone," Connigan pleaded.

"Well, what would you like me to do, ask them in for tea? They're going to die soon anyway. You do know this is for real, don't you? This isn't one of your academic fantasies, or some computer model. John, it's okay. Be proud of what you're doing. And be courageous. You're one of our leaders, we're following you, whether you realize it or not. We're your soldiers, your crusaders, and we're fighting for something very precious.

"In the last hour three animal and plant species have become extinct and the world's population has increased by four thousand. You're the genius, you do the math. It's down to a few decades before it's all over, anyway. The world is choking to death on our poisons. It's bad enough all the magic and mystery are gone from our earth, now mankind is going after its very soul. It's up to us, and you. Science did this, and science will undo this.

"No, I'll take care of anyone who gets in our way," Mr. Natural continued, his voice hardening. "It's not necessarily what I want, but I will do what I must do. And you must do what you must do. We will not fail."

Connigan sat back. Mr. Natural is right, he thought. Crazy people must not get in our way. I will make the necessary modifications.

"Okay, I'll make it work, it's just about done," he said. "Did the amino acids arrive?"

"Everything's in the basement. Someone will take you down to the lab. You rest here. I'll make a big lunch for you."

With that the huge man rose and walked out, leaving Connigan alone in the shadows. He trembled, partly from the realization that the answer to his experiment's problem was starting to gel in his mind. From out of nowhere an idea had materialized. It always seemed to happen like this. He smiled in wonderment as it crystallized and, as if possessed of its own life, found the gap in calculations and fit itself snugly into place. I just found the way, he though, I did it again. I found the way. Soon, I'll go downstairs and plug it all into the computer. First, though, I want to go back.

He closed his eyes.

He was back in the forest. It was a hot, sunny day. Almost immediately the moisture on his face began to dry, as a soft breeze sweetened his lungs. He stood there, basking in the warmth. Then he began to walk in grateful solitude along a secret path.

He brushed away huge green leaves that dangled playfully before him. On each side lay countless flowers. He normally would have sat down amongst them and rest, and perhaps talk to them, but today he had a destination.

In a few minutes he was there. Standing directly in the middle of the path, perfectly upright, with no walls around it, was a door. Constructed from small, thin logs, richly polished, it waited for him. Its very existence seemed illogical. Connigan, the scientist, knew that. But he also knew one even more important thing. The door was magical, and magic, he knew, always trumped science..

Gratefully, he walked up to it, pushed it open and stepped through.

At first glance nothing seemed different, but within seconds he again was aware of the vast transformation.

The leaves were larger and rounder, and the ground was warm and spongy. What fascinated him the mist that was now everywhere, and it lightly bathed everything around him. What Connigan liked most was how the sunbeams played with it as they shot through the trees—everything in their path shimmered.

He walked slowly, taking deep breaths. There wasn't any rush; in fact, the whole concept of schedules had become what he always knew it was, meaningless and superficial. There were no buildings or machines, money or crime, or madness. Everything was at its most basic. Connigan had crossed through several dimensions, the least of which was time.

It's irrelevant, but I wonder how far back I've gone, he mused. My guess is about fifty million years. The dinosaurs are gone, but there aren't any large mammals yet either—I guess they haven't developed yet. There aren't any predators—there's enough here for everything and everyone. I'm in paradise. He took a giant breath and smiled.

He continued along the sliver of a path, until it opened and came upon a small pond surrounded by a carpet of grass. It was one of his favorite places. At its far end, water trickled playfully along smooth rocks. Connigan stood there, nodding approvingly at the beauty before him. He carefully removed his clothes. Then, with his favorite yell, the one he used when he was growing up on the farm, he ran to the edge and dove in.

chapter 19

Ivan leaned against the bars in his cage, thinking for the thousandth time of possible ways to escape. Since his capture in the garage, he had done little more than just sit and stare at his bare surroundings. He had been in prison before, but this was different. Here, he felt like a captured animal.

Out of arms' reach a tall, large man dressed in an ill-fitting white coat looked at him. It seemed to be a near-hourly ritual, and the prisoner barely paid him any mind.

"How are you feeling?" Mr. Natural asked.

"None of your business. You got no right to treat me like this."

"Well, did you have any right to beat those people to death?"

"I didn't do nothing. You got the wrong guy."

The big man smiled. "I very much doubt that."

Ivan violently rattled the cage, snarling at his captor. The sound seemed to completely absorb into the well padded basement room, which had no window.

Mr. Natural walked over to a nearby desk, strewn with paper and various syringes and test tubes. From there he watched patiently, whistling softly. As the outburst waned, Ivan, who now lost track of his days in captivity, began to cry.

"My dear man," his captor began, "You've got to look at the bright side. Your previously miserable life has taken on meaning, perhaps for the first and only time since you were born. Think of it. You've gone from being a dirtball, a loser, a predator, worse, a parasite and scavenger, to being a full participant in the greatest rescue in the history of this world. If everything works out, and it will, I promise you, you will go down in history, unwritten as it will be, as a hero. Unwitting, unwilling, graceless, but a hero nonetheless."

"I don't know what you're talking about."

"You don't have to. As long as we know. That makes it easier on you, Ivan, you can't do anything wrong. Here, have some lunch."

With that, Mr. Natural reached over and picked up a tray. He walked to the cage and slid it through a small opening.

"Hot dogs, ketchup and beer. That's your favorite, isn't it?"

Ivan ignored him. He started stuffing food into his mouth, barely breathing between mouthfuls. He cracked open the beer and washed the food down greedily. After a few minutes he belched and wiped his mouth with a sleeve. He was breathing heavily.

"Man, you just got to let me go," he panted.

"You'll be out soon enough. Here. Have another beer."

"I better be. My people are looking for me."

"Ah, yes, the Death Masters. What a delightful bunch. Your initiation rites include outright murder, don't they? How absolutely wonderful. That's why we chose you and, shall we say—your *brothers*—to experiment on. This part of the operation is practically guilt-free.

"Listen, I've got to tell you something. I'm a vegetarian. Did you know that I even feel bad when I eat cheese, because an animal has been exploited for my sake. But the truth is, I really enjoy testing this stuff on you guys. Somehow it just seems right, when you think about it.

"When Doctor X first told me we'd be testing on human models I was upset. Me? I don't even kill bugs. Just wait and you'll see how right it feels, the good doctor said. And our leader was right, sir, it feels mucho good. Here, have another beer."

"So when am I getting out," Ivan persisted, gulping his food loudly.

Mr. Natural moved closer and peered into his prisoner's face, shining a small light onto it. "Soon enough. Hmm, look at those red dots, you are positively covered. I do believe the bug is going to town on you. Ivan, this may be our last meeting. So, how many wild elephants do you think are left?"

"This a joke?"

"No joke—there's no punch line or anything. I'll even tell you the answer. Maybe a few hundred. A few thousand, if you count zoos and circuses. But the bottom line is that there aren't too many left. It's pretty sad, don't you think?"

Ivan glared at his captor. "One day you are going to die," he said in a low voice.

Mr. Natural looked evenly at him. "Congratulations, you've actually hit a philosophical bulls-eye."

"What?"

"You see, we are *all* going to die. You, and I. Of course you envisioned stabbing me to death and then returning to your seemingly eternal grotesque existence. But the truth is, we're both gonna kick, no matter what we do. It is a little disturbing to think that we'll meet on the other side—I do hope God corrals you and your kind off somewhere far away in the hereafter.

"But I'm digressing. My big concern is, what do I do while I'm here, in this body, with this mind? Should I take the easy, worthless approach like you did? Or should I try to do some good. Ivan, I decided to do good with my life, and even risk it to that end. You may have heard the question, if a tree falls in the middle of an empty forest, does it make a sound? Well if a person lives without having done any good, can that person possibly have had a good life? Think about it. You've maybe an hour left. For God's sake, Ivan, you've lived longer than most of the apostles! Doctor X has, in this small way, legitimized your existence."

"You're a crazy man."

"Possibly … listen, I want to give you some advice. Try to picture a world with uncharted forests, endless meadows filled with wild flowers, and the quiet, haunting desert. It's important to think beautiful thoughts at the very end, if you want my opinion. Good luck, my friend, I'm sure you would have been a much better person in a much different time."

Mr. Natural walked to the door, waved at his captive and gently let himself out.

chapter 20

Connigan resisted the urge to estimate how long he played and splashed in the water. There's no such thing as time anymore, he kept thinking. Or, more precisely, there is no such thing as time yet—clocks, and the humans who invented them, won't make their debut for many millions of years.

He floated on his back, softly paddling across the pond. Several brightly colored birds looked at him from nearby branches.

"I apologize on behalf of all humankind," he said to them. "They used to teach that dinosaurs were horrible monsters. But it turned out that we were the monsters, we were the ones who caused all the real damage. The dinosaurs turned into oil, or at least fertilizer, when they died. We humans just we keep rolling on and on, knocking down everything in our path, leaving nothing behind.

"Looking back, I figure we made two major mistakes. We conquered disease, and we invented science. Darwinian Law didn't stand a chance. That's why I think it's so fitting that the saviors of the planet are none other than a doctor and a scientist."

After a while he left the pool and lay on a patch of willowy grass, letting himself dry off in the warm air. It's so beautiful, he thought. Why do I ever return at all. They all think I'm crazy back there. One day they'll lock me up and I'll be trapped there forever.

"John?"

Connigan looked up. Before him stood Pony. She was the only

person he ever let enter this place. They had even explored it together, going on long walks through the fields, sometimes taking picnics on the hilltops. Pony smiled down at him. She had thick, flowing, golden hair, which glimmered in the sunlight, creating a sensuous halo about her. He stared into her large, gray-blue eyes, which twinkled their welcome. Her tan face was lightly freckled, her teeth were sparkling and her smile was large. She wore a simple white dress, made of thin cotton, which did little to hide her round breasts or her muscular, curved hips.

He was enchanted, as always, by her beauty. All was still and silent about them. The surrounding mist, punctuated by large flowers in every direction, seemed to encase both of them in some kind of mythological portrait. For a brief moment, he felt immortal.

She smiled. "I'm glad you returned."

"No need to worry on that account. I'll always come back. I missed you."

She sat down beside him and touched his leg gently. "I missed you too. I belong to you."

"You knew I'd return, didn't you?"

"Knowing is one thing. Seeing you is another. Please don't leave me again."

"I have a little work to do, there," Connigan said, angrily pointing in an imaginary direction. "My task is to make sure that this paradise never ends."

"If anyone can do it, you can," Pony said, rubbing his belly.

"That feels good," he murmured. "Yes, I can do it. As a matter of fact, a few more days are all I need. And then, when it's all done. I'm going to return and take care of you forever."

"John, I'd love that so much," she said. She moved her hand lower.

He instantly became aroused. He looked up at her longingly.

"First things first, though, huh?" she said coyly. "Maybe I better take care of you."

"I would like that very much."

"Just let me take this off ..."

"Professor?"

"Mmmm ..."

"Professor."

Connigan remained motionless on his chair, his eyes firmly closed. He was moaning softly. One of the men surrounding him nudged him with a finger, his finger sinking into his massive belly. Still, the scientist did not move.

"Leave him alone."

They turned to see Mr. Natural and, beside him, a small, elderly man with long silver hair. The two men walked over to Connigan. Mr. Natural shook his head.

"I guess he's happy that way" he said.

"What is he doing," asked one of the men asked the man with silver hair, known to most outsiders as Jungle Man.

"He's having visions, which will save all of us," Jungle Man replied. "He is sent from the gods."

"Wherever he comes from, he is good for us all," Mr. Natural said. "Soon his medicine will be ready. Very soon. We must guard and protect this man until then."

The huge guard signaled to two of the men. "Stay by him. When he awakens bring him down to the lab. Use the side door. The rest of you, there's a body in cage six that needs to be disposed of."

All the men nodded in agreement and split up. The two men assigned to Connigan patiently sat next to him in the shadows, their heads respectfully turned away, leaving him alone with his visions.

chapter 21

Finkel intently studied his sudoku. Realizing that he didn't have a chance on this one, he decided instead to give Dean another in his new series of lectures, all dedicated to Doctor X. He leaned forward and pointed at Dean with a tongue depressor.

"And let me tell you something else. Everyone makes such a big deal about how beautiful this planet it. 'Ooh, we love it. Ooh we cherish it. Ooh, it's better than a blow job.' And you know what? They're full of doo doo."

Dean, who was sipping some coffee, signing a pile of incomplete charts, nodded absently. Another week had gone by, and the Doctor X issue was fast fading into an amusing anecdote, just another bizarre story in a place filled with them. Even Tannenbaum had shrugged his shoulders and smiled sheepishly when Dean had asked him about the book. Clearly, the world had not come to an end.

Knowing that his friend was on a roll, he let himself play the straight man.

"Okay, why are they full of doo doo?"

"Because you look at any calendar in existence and what pictures do you see next to the month? Slums? Junkyards? The mugger on Bed Five? No. You see pristine mountains with cute little snowcaps, which of course melted three years after they took the picture. And don't forget the mighty pine forests—there's got to be one or two of those left. Or, even more of a joke, cute furry animals that in reality have been driven to the point of extinction.

"In other words, everything that we claim to value about this planet we've done our best to destroy. We are basically romanticizing what we've wiped out. I tell you, it's a sham. All that's left of natural beauty at this point is a few theme parks and some rich people's backyards. And it's going to get worse."

"The great environmentalist has spoken," Dean intoned.

"And that is why I for one am rooting for Doctor X."

"Doctor Finkel, could you come here right away?" Carol gestured from bed three.

"I'll be right back to continue your education," he said to Dean. "Don't leave town or anything. I'm on a roll."

"I'll be here," Dean promised, smiling in spite of himself.

Finkel hurried over to the stretcher. Carol never panicked and she could size up a case better than most physicians. Whenever she asked for help, even politely and calmly as she did now, it was immediately needed. He could tell by the minor subtleties of her tightened forehead and the gentle yet absolute tone of her voice that a disaster was imminent. He braced himself.

"What's up," he asked. As he pulled the curtain he simultaneously looked at Carol, the cardiac monitor and the patient. Before him sitting upright, was a pale, middle-aged woman gasping for breath. Carol was at her side starting an IV, having already put the patient on a face mask giving her pure oxygen. At the other side of the stretcher was the woman's tearful daughter, holding on to her mother's hand.

"Hello, I'm Doctor Finkel. What's going on?"

"She can't breathe," her daughter said worriedly. "It began all of a sudden …"

"What's her pressure," he asked Carol.

"Eighty," Carol said, not looking up.

"Is she going to be all right?" the daughter asked.

Finkel stared at her deeply, and then at the patient.

"Does anything hurt?" he asked her.

"There's something crushing my chest," she gasped. "I can't breathe."

Finkel mind began racing as he quickly but thoroughly spoke with at her, using his experience with over a hundred thousand patients as he watched her move, breathe and answer his questions. He had made his diagnosis before he even touched her. Swiftly he listened to her lungs and heart with a stethoscope, all the while staring at the monitor.

"Start a second line," he told Carol quietly, so as not to be heard by either the patient or her daughter. "Bolus her with amiodarone and titrate dopamine to a systolic of a hundred. She's throwing a million PVC's. Watch the fluid, she's in failure. Let's get a portable chest X-ray and a stat EKG."

"Already ordered," Carol said, holding part of the IV tubing in her clenched teeth.

He turned to the daughter, indulging himself in a slightly longer look than he really had to.

"Why don't you wait outside. I want to examine your mother and begin some treatment."

She nodded nervously and walked away. Carol looked at Finkel with a twinkle in her eye. He moved over to help her with the IV, steadying the woman's cool arm, which like the rest of her was drenched with sweat.

"You seem quite impressed by this young lady," Carol whispered. "You positively undressed her with your eyes."

"Absolutely not," he whispered back indignantly. "That was a purely medical look."

"It looked like a purely medical leer to me."

"I'm wounded. Hey, you're still dating that cop …"

"You're going to talk about that now?"

The patient gasped. Finkel looked at her.

"What's your name?"

"Suzanne," she gasped.

"Suzanne, I want you to hang in there. You'll be fine. Carol, get that pressure over a hundred and start some nitro. And call Respiratory for some BiPAP."

"I'm drowning, help me!" Suzanne gasped.

Finkel's eyes practically bored into her, registering the minutest of subtleties, his mind racing with diagnostic and therapeutic decisions.

Carol watched from the corner of eye with satisfaction. Finkel was regarded as one of the masters, and one of the very few doctors she would let care of her. In the world of nursing that was the highest tribute that could be bestowed upon a physician.

"I bet it's an antero-lateral MI that knocked out a papillary muscle— it's bottomed out her ejection fraction," he told Carol when he was done. At that moment an EKG technician, who had slipped into the room, tore off a hastily completed cardiogram. Finkel looked at it for a second, then at Carol, giving her a smile he reserved for times when he either made a completely accurate diagnosis or when he solved a giant piece of a puzzle.

"It's a biggie," he said quietly, out of the patient's earshot. "Tombstone changes. Get the dopamine started, this may not end well. Have the clerk activate the cath team. Damn, she needs heparin and we don't have an X-ray yet. Excuse me, Suzanne, do you have any medical problems?"

"I had a bleeding ulcer …"

"To heparanize or not to heparinize, that is the question," he said to himself, cutting her off. "Yeah, why not. No guts, no glory."

"Am I going to die," she asked fearfully, struggling to breathe.

"I will take care of you," Finkel said with surprising gentleness, reaching out for her hand.

He turned to the nursing station to shout some orders when something caught his eye. He looked down at the woman. Her eyes began to glow eerily.

"You're losing me," she gasped. "You're losing me."

Instinctively, Finkel knew what had to be done.

"Call a code!" he rasped.

The woman's eyes rolled back and she stopped moving.

"I can't get a pressure," Carol barked out.

Finkel looked up at the monitor.

"V-tach. Shock at 360 joules, now!"

"Don't you want it synchronized?" Harry asked, walking up with a long needle.

"Pulseless V-tach is like V-fib," Finkel said with hurried annoyance, as he broke open the intubation box. "You should know that by now. Start pumping until we get the paddles charged."

Reluctantly, the student obeyed, his face clearly showing regret at having walked ove r to this area. Finkel looked at the woman's daughter, standing down the hall quaking with fear. He yanked the curtain closed and turned back to Carol.

"Is that thing charged yet?"

"Yes."

"Then do it. Back off, Harry!"

Carol squeezed some gel onto the chest, applied the paddles to the chest wall and pressed the button. Electricity shot into the skin, making a little spark. The body spasmed violently, then lay still. At that moment people burst into the cubicle. They all looked up at the monitor. It showed a regular rhythm.

"Check for a pulse," Finkel said calmly.

Carol put a finger to the woman's neck.

"Strong and regular."

"Good, and she's even breathing. We just may be able to hold off on intubation. At least for now."

At that moment the CCU team arrived. The senior cardiology fellow, a petite, attractive woman, stared at the patient, then at Finkel, who winked at her. She smiled back. It was obvious that the two had dated. Carol glared at her.

"Meredith, here's a present for you. Big time MI with shock, cardiac arrest, and a big-time diastolic murmur, which I bet is new. In the mood for a cath?"

The fellow read the chart, then briefly examined the patient.

"No can do, darlin', the lab's down for the next two hours," she said good naturedly. "Keep her down here, on dopamine, heparin, some platelet inhibitor, and we'll call for her, she'll be cool. I'd hold off on a thrombolytic for now ..."

"Put her in the CCU," Carol interrupted. "We're getting killed down here."

"No available beds," Meredith replied coolly. "She'll have to hold down here."

"Bullshit, that's just because it's near the change of shift," Carol snapped. "Bob, I wish we could get away with that crap There are three sick patients waiting for this bed. How long do we have to baby-sit?"

"As long as it takes," Meredith said evenly. She was a slightly built woman who looked far younger than her thirty years. She turned to Finkel and looked at him, her face wearing the hint of a coy pout. "Bob, I'll see what I can do. There's a guy upstairs who's circling the drain. Just hang in there. Pretty please."

"Of course, take your time," Finkel effused.

Carol looked away furiously.

At that moment a voice over the loudspeaker began its familiar boom.

"Attention please, attention please, Doctor Heart, CCU. Doctor Heart, CCU."

Those were the words, so as not to disturb patients or visitors, signaling a full arrest. Carol looked at Julie, who had walked over. They nodded at each other and smiled.

Meredith turned to Finkel and whispered. "So, you're in luck. You guys will have that bed soon. We gotta go. Hey, call me."

Then she and her team were gone.

Finkel left the cubicle and walked over to the daughter. She was trembling uncontrollably and cringed as he approached.

"She's okay, she's okay," he said soothingly. "I think she'll do just fine."

The young woman began to rock with quiet sobs. At that minute an admitting clerk walked over.

"Honey, could you give us some information about your mom?"

The clerk led her to a nearby desk. The daughter, her face wet with tears, looked at Finkel and mouthed the words "thank you." Finkel waved at her. Then he turned and walked back to the station. He sat down and returned to the puzzle, hoping that the commotion had loosened up some answers in his brain.

Dean was still at his seat. He glanced at Finkel and chuckled.

"So big guy, what do you have to say for yourself?"

Finkel looked at him.

"Where else can you save lives and find romance at the same time? I love emergency medicine."

Both doctors burst out laughing.

chapter 22

Another week had gone by. For Dean, the days blended into one another. He had by now worked eighteen consecutive twelve hour days, almost all in the Big Room, an unheard of and technically illegal phenomenon in a field where even five consecutive was considered a burnout pace. He worked furiously, seeing nearly forty patients a day. He dazzled his colleagues with his efficiency and awed them with his intensity. It got to the point where they started asking him for advice, even the great Finkel.

Dean barely acknowledged his near-frenzied pace. The wilder and more chaotic the ER became, the more relaxed he seemed to become. He practically planted himself in the Big Room and he couldn't seem to get enough. Normally, even the most battle-hardened ER doctor would last only a few days in a row here, it being too bloody, too catastrophic, too close to death. Dean seemed to flourish here, and when his shifts ended he practically had to be persuaded to leave. It was as if he was afraid to emerge from this grotesque but violently predictable chaos deep in the inner city.

Finally, Finkel asked him why he seemed to like "living" in the ER so much.

"You really want to know?"

"Yeah, you've been so working so much we don't get together anymore. It used to be fun having a few drinks after work. What gives? Just don't get too heavy. I'm not very good at empathy or anything to do with feelings. That's why I got into emergency medicine to being with."

Dean couldn't help but smile. Finkel was the perfect foil. He had the air of a bartender leaning over the counter—all he needed was a washcloth in one hand.

"Okay, here goes. Stop me if you get creeped out. I'm really getting sort of depressed. Not dysfunctional or anything, but well, nothing seems to be fun anymore. I stay here because I can't find a reason to leave. I'm way past the halfway point in my life, way past, judging from my family genetics, and there just isn't much to show. A wasted marriage, no kids, not too much money, not too much of anything. I don't think I've even been in love—during those fourteen years the best we managed was 'like', and that was pretty rare.

"Guys my age should be buying birthday presents, anniversary presents, mowing their lawns, arguing with contractors, going to family get-togethers, I don't know, something. I'm still here, I haven't changed. I'm doing the exact same stuff I was doing fifteen years ago, I'm just a little better at it now. I've come full circle and I'm back to nowhere. Somewhere, something went wrong. I can't figure out what, or why."

Finkel bit his upper lip, feeling sorrow for his friend and anger at himself for not knowing what to say.

"I'm pretty much alone, lately," Dean continued. "I walk alone, I drink wine alone, I sleep alone. And now, of course, I'm forty six, and have gray hairs everywhere. I'm too old to fantasize about half the women I meet. And, in thirty years, give or take, I'll be dead. That's it in a nutshell."

"So you come to the ER to get away from it all?" Finkel asked, as if he were comparing notes.

"No, I come here because it's all I have. There's nothing for me on the outside. The Big Room fills me up, gives me something to do. It keeps me one step ahead of the blues. Until I can figure how to stop feeling sorry for myself, I'm afraid to stop."

"You do know that things aren't that bad," Finkel said.

"Of course. Maybe it's all some male menopausal crap. But you know things are bad when you read that crazy guy's book and start agreeing with him about destroying the world."

"No, no no, don't tell me you're still involved with that. Dean, that was yesterday's joke. It's over, man, put it to rest."

"I made a copy before I turned it in," Dean whispered conspiratorially. " Fink, it's interesting stuff. I've checked out his theories and proofed his equations—they're right on the money."

"Dean, do you want this 'stuff' to be true?"

"Bob, the world is going to hell in a hand basket, and we both know it."

"Dean, please don't make me worry about you …"

"Doctor Miller, could you come over here?" an aide said, gesturing from Bed Nine. "Julie said to come right away."

"Be right there," Dean said. He shook hands with Finkel. "Thanks for listening."

"Anytime. And stop with the end of the world stuff. And listen, while you're there, check out Julie. She is looking hot, and she's been saying some very positive things about you. Forget this Doctor X, that woman has the cure for what's ailing you. Know what I mean?"

"Yeah."

Dean walked towards the room, squeezing past several stretchers. Julie was waving to him from Bed Nine. Finkel's right, he thought, she's gorgeous.

Soon he was at the stretcher; on it lay an unconscious woman in her late thirties. Next to her was her boyfriend. He was badly overweight, which was made all the more obvious by his painfully tight denim pants and jacket—his stomach practically exploded over his waistline. What was left of his long hair had been pulled back into a ponytail, and through his bushy beard one could see gaps among brownish teeth. He shuffled nervously on old, pointed boots.

"About an hour ago I was dogging her really good. Didn't think anything about it, she likes it that way. Then it was like something ripped inside her. She fainted before the ambulance came. Oh yeah, she's a little pregnant. I'm going out for a cigarette."

With that, he turned and walked out of the room. Dean and Julie were alone with the pale woman, who lay motionless before them.

"Can you believe that?" snapped a nearby resident. She had been applying a splint to an ankle fracture. "How crude can people get? It's disgusting. Dogging her!"

"I don't know, it depends on who's doing it, right hon'?" Julie said, winking at Dean. "I can think of worse things ... wow, look at the tattoos on this lady. I wonder which one of the names on her ass is that guy?"

"So, it sounds good to you, huh?" Dean said, trying to sound casual. He desperately fought back a growing tightness in his chest.

"Like I said, it all depends," Julie said, looking evenly at him. "You know what I mean?"

Dean forced himself to keep breathing. With effort he forced his attention to the patient before him. Within a minute he had made his diagnosis.

"This has got to a ruptured ectopic," he said. "Get this lady ready for the OR, and have the secretary page OB stat."

"Why do you think it's an ectopic?" Julie asked while starting an IV.

"She's pregnant, with vaginal bleeding and sudden onset of pain. Now she's in shock and has a distended abdomen. And by the way," he turned to the resident, who was walking away. "This was inevitable. Her boyfriend just rushed it along."

"I know, I know," she said grudgingly. "It's just his attitude."

"He was a little uncouth, Dean," Julie said. "I'm sure you'd phrase it much more tenderly, right?"

"But of course," Dean said, trying to sound cool.

Julie inserted a plastic tube into the woman's nose and threaded it into her stomach. She was across the stretcher from him and leaning forward as she worked, the front of her scrub shirt pulling away from her, exposing slightly more than a hint of her breasts. Dean couldn't help but look. Julie looked up at him, smiling.

"You like what you see?"

"It certainly is a temptation," he said nervously.

"That's the idea, Dean," she said quietly. "There's more."

"Can I say something un-medical and not related to this case ..."

"Talk to me, Dean."

"I'd really like to see you ..."

"I'm really glad, it's time," Julie said, reaching into her shirt's breast pocket. She extracted a piece of paper and put it in Dean's hand. "Come on over after your shift. We can listen to music or something."

"Or something," Dean said, using his last shred of mental energy to maintain an aura of stability. "I'll be there."

He was grateful when two tired looking residents walked up, dressed in surgical scrubs. They looked at the comatose woman in disgust.

"Dean, you're killing us," the senior one said. "Every time you work you load us up. What gives now?"

Quickly Dean presented the case to them. Grumbling, both nodded and began wheeling the stretcher to the elevator.

"Nice work. We just might have a save on this one," the senior resident said, his voice trailing. "But do me a favor ... please go home. I'm dead."

Dean grinned. That casual-sounding mark, even from a resident, was the stuff ER physicians prized. They traditionally toiled in near anonymity and were required to be perfect; they only seemed to be recognized when they made a mistake.

He nodded goodbye at Julie and decided to take a break, before he ruined everything by making an ass of himself. He started down the hall to get some coffee in the staff lounge. He was digging in his pocket for the key, when he felt a gentle tap on his shoulder. Turning around, he found himself looking into the face of Mr. Natural. Before he could stop himself, he started violently.

"Relax, Doc, I don't bite," he said genially.

"You surprised me. Did you follow me here?"

"Not at all, good buddy, I was here ... you walked by me. You must have a lot of stuff on your mind."

"Nothing out of the ordinary. Now if you will excuse me ... wait a minute, I was curious, have you seen your friend Connigan lately?"

Dean detected the slightest narrowing of the guard's eyes.

"Him? Nah. He's probably wandering around somewhere. It's a big city, you know? Why do you ask?"

"Just curious. I've thought about him from time to time."

"Well, if I do see him, I'll say 'hi' for you. Okay? Take care, Doc, nice talking to you."

The large man went toward the ER and disappeared. Dean was angry at having forced the conversation and using Connigan's name. The whole incident had disturbed him, particularly the guard's role in it. He forced it all from his mind and, looking around him, went into the lounge for some coffee.

chapter 23

"Hey, look at this," Ehler called out from Bed Two.

Dean, Finkel and Helen walked over. It was at the end of another long shift, and they were winding down. Ehler was standing beside an unconscious man lying motionless on a stretcher, who clearly looked as if he had come from the streets. The doctor absently palpated his abdomen while they approached.

"Check this out," he said again.

They looked down, and within a second each recognized the problem.

"A generalized petechial rash," Helen said. "What's the platelet count."

"I just got it back from the lab. They had to run it through twice," Ehler said. "It's under a thousand."

"That's pretty low, even for a booze hound," Finkel said, impressed. "Is he on chemo or something? I don't expect guys like this to be normal, but this is ridiculous."

"I agree with you," Ehler said. "I got his old chart and he doesn't have much of a medical background. His platelet count was actually normal last month. He doesn't even have a big liver. His hemoglobin is eight. But the really scary thing is that his white count is six hundred. All lymphocytes. "

"No neutrophils?" Dean asked incredulously. "The lab didn't find one?"

116

"Not a one. They even recalibrated their machine and ran it again. They thought there was a short circuit somewhere."

"His bone marrow just completely shut off," Finkel murmured.

Finkel's phase bothered Dean, but he couldn't figure why. He shrugged it off.

"What are you doing for him?" he asked Ehler.

"For now I'm treating him for septic shock. He's cultured up and I'm running in some vancomycin, gentamycin and cephtriaxone. I'm also going to transfuse him fresh frozen plasma and platelets. He needs a bed in the ICU fast. With his numbers, if you so much as look at him the wrong way, he's going to die."

"Nice case," Finkel said. "I think I'd wash my hands after this one."

"An overwhelming viral infection could do this, don't you think?" Dean said, staring at the body. Finkel looked at him sourly.

"Sure, although there was no prodrome. According to witnesses he was feeling fine and just sort of stopped dead in his tracks," Ehler said. "Of course, a very rapid acting pathogen could potentially ..."

"Maybe he was poisoned," Helen said.

"Maybe he was," Ehler replied. "This could be anything. Look at that arrhythmia on the monitor—whatever is going on is even affecting his heart. This guy is literally shutting down in front of us."

Something stirred deep within Dean, making him uneasy. Then a string of words dangled before his mind, something he had recently read: "*I will stop all motion deep within us. I will shut down our very cores and we will begin to freeze from the inside out.*"

"It's as if this man was shut off like a switch," he said.

"What are you talking about?" asked Helen.

"Nothing, nothing, forget what I said."

"Wait, we had a deal," Finkel said. "I stop nominating Connigan for sainthood and you stop believing in his fairy tales."

"Okay, okay, forget it."

A medical student walked over, a liver biopsy tray in his hand. He leaned over to look in the dying man's face. With a finger he pulled down his lower eyelid.

"Do you think the shpos is going to kick soon?" he asked.

"I'd be careful, he's probably teeming with alien organisms," Finkel whispered back. "Overwhelming sepsis, know what I mean?"

"Holy shit," the student muttered, his eyes widening. "That's the second one in two days."

"What do you mean?" Ehler asked.

"Well, I had just come back from grand rounds, it was on new therapies for psoriasis. Who cares about that stuff. I mean, it was boring …"

"Get to the point," Dean interrupted with annoyance.

"Anyway, my first patient when I got here, he was just like this. He also had a big subdural hematoma, from being punched. Know why he bled so much? He had two thousand platelets. And no white count. He died this morning in the ICU. I assisted on the case last night and even got to intubate. Oh shit, and I touched him."

The student suddenly pulled his hand back as if it had been shocked—he held his finger away from his body, looking at it as if it were contaminated.

"Did he say anything about what happened?" Dean asked.

"Yeah, before he went out he talked a lot," the student murmured uneasily, still looking at his finger. "Can I be excused and wash this?"

"Did he say anything about drinking strange concoctions, any recent travel …"

"Well, he'd been drinking. He did say that he and a few friends stole a case of whisky off the back of a truck a few nights before. It was funny because the owners of the truck weren't too far off and were watching them. He said it was almost like they were waiting for them to steal it, and they didn't even chase after them."

"Almost like they were setting them up to drink the stuff," Dean mused. "Anything else?"

"No except that the guys from the truck looked strange, foreign, like out of the travel shows you see on television, when they go to the jungle. I swear, that's what he said."

"Very interesting," Dean said.

"There it is, Dean, your conspiracy at work," Finkel said. "The First Worlders of the jungle are going to war against the Second Worlders of modern society, but first they're sparring with the Third Worlders, their bastard children. Sort of like training for the main bout, know what I mean?"

"Let him finish," Helen said. She looked quizzically at the student. "What else did he say?"

"That's pretty much it. He was only conscious for a few minutes. He didn't say much more."

"Go on, go wash your finger," Finkel said, dismissing him. "Be careful the next time a resident lets you do a procedure he was supposed to do, it's usually a dump. And be careful picking your nose."

The medical student raced off, holding his arm straight up as he ran.

Dean looked at Finkel.

"There's obviously a connection between the two patients, don't you think?"

"Two dirtballs hit the dust, and you think some avenging eco-angel is on the move. Nice imagination. Come on, let's get a drink. We can toast to the memory of Maximo the Caveman, who is now extinct."

"What happened to Max?" Dean asked.

"They found him dead in some alley. Covered with bruises. Someone probably beat the crap out of him. It's not like he had any shortage of enemies."

"What was his platelet count," Dean asked anxiously. Bad feelings within him were stirring.

"We'll never know. He was already dead, extremely dead, and went straight to the morgue. Dean, he was the king of the shpos, it's a miracle he lasted this long. He had a million things wrong with him, and he abused every substance known to man. Remember, when you hear the thunder of beating hooves, don't think of zebras. I'm sure the Caveman died of, well it's stretch calling them 'natural causes', but certainly I sure none of this Doctor X weirdness ... wait, why are we even having this conversation?"

"Why didn't they do an autopsy."

"Because they probably were afraid to touch him," Finkel said with exasperation. He gripped his friend's forearm. "Dean, you're killing me.

Come on, let's get that drink. You're having a double. No, make that a triple."

As Dean left the ER, being gently guided by his good friend Finkel, he couldn't help but recall, over and over, one phrase from Connigan's book.

I will make everything stop; nothing will stand in my way.

chapter 24

"And who do we have here ... ah yes, our good friend Jack. Oh my goodness, you poor man, you look like you're starving."

Mr. Natural touched both hands to his chest and made the saddest face he could.

Jack eyed his captor coldly. He'd been a prisoner for what had seemed forever; there were no clocks or windows and he knew neither the time nor the place. He knew only that he was in a small room locked in a large cage, furnished only with a bare mattress, a small commode and several bottles of water. Aside from a table opposite him outside his cage, which was laden with vials of different colored fluids, the place was totally stark, the only contact with the world this big, strange man, who periodically made visits, writing things down on a clipboard. He was starving.

"How are you feeling, Jack? Wait a minute, that sounds too formal. I mean, we've known each other for quite a while now. Would you mind if I called you 'Jackie?' Why not, we're old friends by now. So, how are you feeling, Jackie?"

"Let me out of here and you'll see how I'm feeling."

"Now, now, no need to be churlish. I let you keep that camel hair coat from your elevator caper, didn't I? Come on, let's put on our happy face. I have a great surprise for you. Ready? I have a snack."

With that Mr. Natural reached into his pocket and pulled out a bag. He pushed it through the cage.

"We made it just for you. You'll love it."

After a moment's pause, Jack ripped the bag open and pulled out what seemed to be an empty hot dog bun. It was slathered in ketchup and relish. Nearly beside himself with hunger he raised it to his mouth. He looked up at the guard.

"There's nothing in it," he growled.

"Silly me, I forgot. Stick the bun outside the cage."

Jack did as he was told. Mr. Natural stuck Jack's lunch inside it. Just before cramming it in his mouth he looked down at it. He literally jumped at the sight. His face twisted wildly. He was staring at the finger he had cut off.

"You fucker," he hissed, hurling the object at the guard, who ducked and turned to watch it bounce off a wall.

"I figured you were the type who enjoyed finger foods," Mr. Natural said, with a half-smile. "Oh well, there's no accounting for taste, as they say.

"Oh, please don't be like that. I'm sorry the way things have turned out. Listen, I have great news. First, you can have a cookie for dessert. We made it special, just for you. And there are no body parts in it. Second, we won't even be needing you after tonight."

With that, he pulled a large chocolate chip cookie out of his pocket and rolled it towards his prisoner. After looking at it haughtily, as if snubbing it, Jack pounced and pushed the cookie into his mouth, nearly inhaling it in his rush.

"What a great appetite," Mr. Natural remarked with admiration. "You must have made your mother very happy indeed at the dinner table. I bet you loved your mother, right? Of course, I heard a vicious rumor, from someone who was actually quite close to where you are at this very moment. He had the nerve, the gall, the impudence if you will, to claim that you once mugged your mother for drug money, and that because of it she died a heart attack. Rumors, aren't they terrible? I'd never talk to him again, no, better than that, I'd call a lawyer. Oh, what's the matter, Jackie, you look like you've seen a ghost."

Jack slammed into the bars of his cage, reaching wildly for the other man.

"I'll kill you!" he screamed.

"I know you don't mean that," the guard said evenly. "You're just upset because you're a free spirit, and now you're in a cage. Things will be fine soon. Real soon."

Jack looked around. He's lying, he thought. I gotta get out of here. There's got to be a way. There's got to be an opening.

He heard Mr. Natural turn to leave. Think fast, he thought. Think fast.

He made a violent gagging motion, clutched his chest and crashed into the ground. With half closed eyes he saw his captor turn around and walk back to the cell, peering at him. Come on, man, come closer, come on.

"Oh my goodness, the prisoner has fainted," Mr. Natural said, his eyes widening. "Oh no, he looks like he's really sick. Jackie, you okay? Jack?"

Jack lay still, waiting for his chance.

"What am I going to do?" Mr. Natural said aloud in a worried tone. "I'm responsible for this man, I can't let anything happen. Wait, I've got it. I'll go into the cage and see if he needs first aid. Then I'll call an ambulance. Where are those keys ... ahh, there they are."

With that the large man put a key into the cage's lock and noisily opened the door. Silently, without making a move, Jack tensed his body, preparing to strike. The guard walked over to him.

"Goodness gracious, I hope he's all right," he murmured, bending over his prisoner. The guard gently poked his prisoner in the back. "Hello there, how are you? Is everything all right?"

He leaned over the prostrate man, craning his neck to look into his face.

Now! thought Jack. *Get him!*

But nothing happened.

Get him! he screamed to himself. *Get up and get him!*

Nothing happened.

He became sick with horror as he realized that he could not move a muscle. Even opening his eyelids was impossible, and he noticed how hard it was to breathe. He wanted to shout with fear, but he couldn't open his mouth. Uncontrollably, his bowels and bladder loosened. More than anything he wanted to open his eyes and escape the drowning darkness—a scene from his distant past flew before him, of his father holding his head under water in a dark room—but his lids would not open. He was totally helpless, and berserk with terror.

"Gee, we've done a number one and a number two all at once," Mr. Natural calmly said, sitting beside his victim, crossing his legs. "Jack, that's a number three. Who says you haven't accomplished anything with your life—aside from giving the police something to do, that is. Not me. In fact, you've done something really important. You've completed our experiments. The whole thing works! Isn't that great?

"You see, you used to be a loser scumbag, despite apparently being quite intelligent. I hear you read a lot, and even spout Latin on occasion. Quite impressive. At the end of the day, however, you were just another sociopath who contributed to the decline of the world. Well, good news, you've graduated from being part of the problem to being part of the solution. Congrats are in order.

"With all due respect, Jack, you really were part of the problem. Did you say something? Oh, that was just a little more number two, for a moment I thought you were demurring. Where was I ... oh yes, not only were you and your friends a part of the problem, you were not an aberration—you were a natural by-product of modern times. Getting rid of you would only open a spot for one or two more of you. That's why we had to go after the very system that spawned you.

"And don't even get me started on the environment, I could talk you to, well, death. The redwoods are gone, the rain forest is nearly gone, the glaciers are gone. For goodness sake, you have to go a zoo to see most anything. But you know something? What bothers me most is that the mystery is all gone. The entire world is now a tiny, flat dot. You can stand in the middle of the desert, on top of a mountain, or be rafting down a river, and you can get a phone call from someone trying to sell you insurance. Isn't there something obscene about that?"

For the briefest moment Mr. Natural's voice cracked. Jack concentrated on breathing.

"I tell you, Jack, I sometimes wonder if we have the right to do all this. Hurting something doesn't come easy to me, in that way you're tougher than me. But then I look at a small cluster of trees or I see a picture of a whale or a tiger, and I get mad, and I find the strength to do this. You know, it's their world, too. And we used to share it. There's enough for everyone, Jack, you stinking piece of shit. Maybe after you and your ilk are gone we can start all over again, and maybe we'll get it right this time.

"You didn't know it, but you have the virus, and were going to die. We are terminating you before you get very sick. This is actually more humane, which is something you probably couldn't relate to. And don't feel bad that we picked you. You were bad news, amigo, and were just going to get into more trouble, a few more fucks, a few more highs, a few more bad deeds. If anything, we saved you from a few more million years in hell."

Jack began to suffocate. He remained motionless, ironically, in the very position he himself had selected. Mr. Natural watched him turn color. After a few minutes he lifted a wrist and then dropped it, watching it slap onto the floor.

"Good luck, my dirtball friend, *ab imo pectore*, from the bottom of my heart. I wonder what you would have been like if you had grown up in another time and place. You could have been a great man, we'll never know. The way it stands now, I figure you have a lot of roasting to do in the next life."

He stared at the lifeless body for a while, then got up and pushed a button on the wall.

"Clean out this room," he said impassively. "Activate the shutdown procedure and make preparations to leave. We're now entering the final phase."

Mr. Natural exited the room and walked down the basement hall. As he walked by each room he saw well-rehearsed activity, as men flawlessly moved into action, beginning to pack boxes, destroy records and pour chemicals down drains. His heart started to race in excitement. It's really going to happen, he thought, the Final Crusade is about to begin. Nothing can stop us now.

Mr. Natural walked into Connigan's room without knocking and sat down at the end of his bed. Connigan was sleeping soundly, on his side; his snores filled the air. Mr. Natural stared at the naked man in amazement. How does he get through the day, with all that fat. No muscles at all, no grace, no coordination. But that mind, that dazzling mind. I'm glad Doctor X discovered him. This crazy professor will be out savior, providing he doesn't bring the police down on our heads first.

"Wake up," he said, tapping the scientist's feet. The large man started and instantly opened his eyes. He looked at Mr. Natural.

"John, it works. Congratulations. Prepare the materials. Doctor X estimates we need a total of two kilograms, in two separate containers. The virus particles go in one and the starter enzymes in the other. We'll keep it nice and simple. We're breaking up shop here and going to the various safe houses. You'll be taken to one and you can finish there."

"Then we're going to start it soon?"

"When can you get things ready?"

Connigan looked down, making calculations in his head. "We'll make the deadline. But we're falling short on vaccines. I'll need about a week."

"That's way too long. Remember the little book you left behind? We could have moved the target date back, but now we can't. We stick to the planned release date. Luckily, you made that breakthrough, otherwise it would have been close. But we still can't waste a second, John. That book's out there. They're going to find us."

Connigan made a face. He sucked mucous loudly through his nose and swallowed. Mr. Natural stared at him with disgust.

"I wish there were more vaccines," Connigan said, scratching his nose. "Most have already been mailed out. I have about six hundred left, and you want most of those for additional worldwide distribution ..."

"We'll be sending them out tomorrow," Natural interrupted. "We have people waiting for them and we will keep our word."

"That doesn't leave me much, considering the doubling time of nearly twenty hours. It's pure math; I need more time."

"Do the best you can. I guess some people just won't make the cut, and that's too bad. You're certain the bacteria in this vaccine reproduce in fresh water?"

"That's actually quite easy," the scientist said. "This primitive strain thrives under very crude conditions, and they are prolific. Put them in their dry state on a piece of paper, under a stamp, mail the letter, and throw the letter in some warm water, even a pond or lake. It's as simple as that. A few days later drink the water. The only side effect may be a little diarrhea. The ones who received the scratch vaccine won't even get that."

"Good, very good. You know, it took us a year to select the protected areas and make the contacts. Half of those people still don't fully understand what it's all about, but they'll go along. We have Jungle Man to thank for that. Everyone trusted him. Two days ago we used up thirty doses for more of his people. We promised them protection, and we made good on it."

"Then you've left me with that much less to work with."

"So be it," Mr. Natural said casually, stretching his huge frame as he stood up. "Keep up the good work, big guy. In a few days we're saving the world."

Mr. Natural patted Connigan on the leg and walked out. The scientist rolled onto his back. He knew it was time to get up and start working, but it felt delicious just laying there. The room was totally still. Very softly, very gently, he heard a rushing sound. It became louder, and began to envelope him ...

He was back in the forest now, under the ancient sun. He walked on a well worn path known only to him. Moving effortlessly, he brushed past large, friendly leaves, heading for the clearing. I'm making good time, he thought, there's plenty of sunlight left. I hope Pony is there. She makes every day a holiday.

Along the way he stopped to examine the flowers, which abounded in all shapes and colors. He touched a few in wonderment, astonished as always at their total perfection. He was in no rush. There was no danger in this world, no predators, animal or human. It would be millions of years before mankind's lightning ride off the cliff, he thought. For now, the world was in total harmony, and he had no fear of rumbling trucks or overhead planes interrupting the sweet song of nature.

This is the real world, he thought, not that angry, crowded cesspool I used to live in. This is the real thing. Soon, I'll never have to leave it.

He resumed walking, and soon broke out of the wooded path. Before him was small, circular clearing, sliced through the towering walls of green all around. It was carpeted by a bed of fallen leaves. Except for an occasional whistle or chirp from the brightly colored birds, and the refreshing rustle the leaves in the soft breeze, all was quiet and peaceful.

In the very center of the scene sat Pony, a basket next to her. She's so beautiful, Connigan thought. Her eyes contain the secret of the universe, and when I make love to her I truly know the meaning of all existence. The honor of my life has been that she has chosen me.

Pony got up and walked over. She touched his arm. As always, she wore a simple, hand woven dress. It rested gently on her breast and hips.

"I'm glad you returned," she said.

"You knew I would."

"Seeing you makes me feel so happy. Are you hungry? I brought food."

She led him to her spot. They sat down on a white cotton blanket. Connigan held onto her hand and looked tenderly at her. In the old world he would have been frozen with shyness and fear in the presence of this dazzling woman.

"Pony, soon I'll be able to stay forever. A few more days, some minor adjustments and all the solutions will be ready. Even now I think we could do it. In two or three days it's a guarantee."

Pony touched the side of his face. "That would be very nice. Sometimes I'm afraid you'll be stopped and I'll never see you again."

Connigan trembled. "It won't happen, they're protecting me. We're pretty much done, now we're making extra vaccines. We're going to spare selected people all over the world."

"Who are they?"

"Well, they're making the final decisions, but they basically include original peoples and the best of the new ones. We're not worried about the re-emergence of technology—it should disappear in a matter of weeks. Organized civilization will simply implode. It's actually quite fragile. Take away fuel, medicine and electricity and you have total, permanent, collapse. We figure on an eventual post-epidemic census of less than fifty million, and they will live primal, simple, natural lives."

Pony smiled. "How lovely," she said. "It's almost too good to be true. We'll go back to the essence. John, you're such a hero. You've rescued the world, the entire planet. I'll worship you for the rest of my life."

Connigan looked down, blushing. Then they both laughed. Pony was the first to speak.

"Can I fix you something to eat?"

"I'd like to start with a little sugar," he replied, secretly delighted that he had gotten this long practiced line out without a flaw.

He leaned over and kissed her. She wrapped her arms around him and kissed back passionately. He gradually lowered her down to the soft ground. Silently, gracefully, they shed their clothes and embraced again. Pony was exquisitely responsive. When he timidly put his hand between her legs she made a little sound of pleasure. His sensations at that moment were that of sheer exhilaration. I've finally made it to the top of the world, he thought. They held onto each other, filled with passion, as they made love deep into the primeval afternoon in the secret, long-lost world.

chapter 25

On a Friday morning, on his twentieth consecutive day of work, Dean recoiled in horror at a woman convulsing before him. She had presented with an asthmatic attack, and was rapidly deteriorating before him. Her seizures were violent; she nearly fell off the stretcher, every muscle in her body jerking wildly.

Dean covered his face with his hands, out of fear for the woman, and out of guilt and anger at himself—he had committed a terrible mistake. Carol stood several feet away, staring at him disapprovingly.

"Holy shit, what's going on? Finkel asked, walking quickly over. He looked up at the cardiac monitor. "V-Tach. What gives."

"I gave her some IV epinephrine for her asthma," Dean mumbled. "I pulled it out of the multi-dose vial and messed up the dose. She got at least three milligrams. I pushed it on my own, so a nurse wasn't around to catch it. God, I feel so bad."

"It happens," Finkel said, taking control of the case. "Carol, give her a hundred of lidocaine, two of lorazepam, and prepare to shock. These arrhythmias can be a bitch. I'll try to hold off on labetalol, considering the asthma. Oh yeah, draw up some succinylcholine, I'm tubing her. Does anyone have any gum?"

He turned to Dean, who seemed stunned. "Don't worry about this," he said gently. "They usually come out of this. No one will even know. Dean, that was a rookie error, what were you thinking about?"

"I don't know, she wasn't responding to the basic stuff. My mind

130

was spinning. There was an IV-epinephrine/magnesium study in the *Journal* last month."

"I read that article, too. It's a piece of crap."

"I know. Bob, I feel so bad."

"This is from you working so much. You eventually had to mess up somewhere. Your batting average is still pretty high, if you ask me. Wait outside for a second."

Finkel closed the curtain. Carol ran over with three syringes, each filled with clear fluid. Five minutes later they motioned for Dean to enter. The patient lay still, breathing slowly and evenly through a breathing tube hooked into a mechanical respirator.

"I thought this couldn't happen to me," Dean whispered.

"It can happen to anyone," Finkel responded, looking all the while at the monitor above the bed. "Oxygen saturation is a hundred. And look, she's back in sinus rhythm. At least for now. Dean, we are human, despite what you think, and despite what our patients think. And humans make mistakes, especially when they're tired. And since you are both human and tired, you just made a beauty. Big, fucking, deal."

Meredith, the CCU fellow, was in the ER and saw the commotion. She walked over and conferred with Finkel a few feet away, while Dean stared at his patient helplessly. The two doctors then burst into laughter, and they returned to their distraught colleague.

Meredith smiled at Dean. "Listen, I'll take her up to the unit. It'll be a piece of cake. She'll be kissing our hand by the time she leaves. No one will ever know. If I know you, you didn't even chart this stuff yet."

"No, not yet."

"Get some coffee, Dean, we'll take care of it."

Numbly, he walked away. The rest of the ER seemed oblivious to what had just happened. He sat down heavily in a chair at the nursing station. After a few minutes he lay his head down on the desk before him and drifted into an uneasy sleep.

There was a tap on his shoulder. He looked up groggily. Julie was smiling at him. For a moment he didn't know where he was.

"Boy, I didn't know I burnt you out so much," she said with a wink. "You sure burnt me out."

"I didn't realize I was so tired. Yeah, maybe this is all your doing," he said, forcing a smile.

They both laughed. Several nights before they had spent hours in each other's arms, wrapped in a mutual sexual frenzy. Dean initially had been petrified entering her apartment, barely able to walk, much less make conversation. Julie seemed to sense this, and kissed him the moment she realized his helplessness. Her tenderness worked. Dean had been so starved for affection that he seemed nearly superhuman—he astonished both of them with his passion.

Julie's mysterious significant other, it turned out, was not a consultant at all, but rather a man in organized crime, and he was completing the end of a one year prison sentence, for what Dean deliberately did not ask. Julie had gently implied this would be a one time only fling. Dean was secretly grateful. He and Julie really had nothing in common and relatively little to talk about, so in his own way he was glad that this time with her had turned out to be just a brief but glorious adventure. They parted as good friends. He couldn't help but recall the mutual sullenness that usually followed lovemaking during his marriage.

"You okay?" Julie asked, cocking her head.

"Well, I'm better now that I see you. But if you want to know the truth, this has not been one of my better days."

"Then I hope this is just a coincidence, but I have a message. Dr. Tannenbaum wants to see you in his office right away."

With that, Julie blew him a kiss and walked away.

chapter 26

Tannenbaum was at his desk, looking into a large, leather-bound text when Dean walked in. Dean knew this was a pose—everyone who ever walked into that office reported that the chief was looking into that book when they entered. The only one not in on the joke was Tannenbaum himself, who feigned mild surprise when Dean approached. He gently closed the book and smiled, and gestured Dean to sit down.

He was a big man, appearing tough and academic, grizzled and intelligent, all at the same time. He seemed to fit the public's fancy as to what a big city chief should look like, and as such was adored by the media. His doctors occasionally grumbled that they would do all the dirty work and that he would get all the attention, but most begrudged him his glory—Tannenbaum had paid his dues and had done so when ER doctors were held in ridicule. More importantly, he was one of the reasons why emergency medicine was rising in prestige, having fashioned a top-flight, internationally known department. The staff doctors all knew that their own stock went up every time their boss appeared before a camera.

"How are you, Dean?"

"Fine, thanks," Dean eyed the older man warily, wondering what he knew.

"I've noticed a significant increase in your hours lately. Is there some problem?"

"I don't know, is there some problem?"

"Don't misunderstand. Your work has been acceptable. But you must understand that I'm concerned."

"Concerned?" Dean asked, stung that his work had been described only as 'acceptable.' "May I ask the reason?"

"It's not about the quality of your work, but rather, the enormous amount of hours. Why so many?"

"Well, no one said I couldn't. And I felt like working, and there were available shifts ..."

"Sometimes it's possible to overdo things, isn't it?" his chief asked softly.

Dean could feel himself starting to tremble. "It didn't seem like too much," he mumbled.

"Don't take this the wrong way, but it is. You'll burn out for sure, and at this rate, soon. That's the big danger in our field, burnout. You're too good and you've got too much of a future. I can't let this happen. I'll ask again, is there a problem?"

Dean sat there. He had paused for too long, and his fatigue and sadness, which had been stalking him, seemed to crash into him from behind. Uncontrollably, tears welled up in his eyes. He wanted to talk, but was fearful and embarrassed. He just sat there.

Tannenbaum briefly went back to his large book, pretending not to notice Dean's distress. Without looking up, he began to speak.

"When I was younger, I lost my wife in a fire. Of course I was working when she died. You have no idea how guilty I felt. It almost destroyed me. To ease the pain I began to work, even harder than you are now. I worked like a dog, and then I killed someone. A real botch. Dean, I fucked up."

Dean visibly started at the word. Tannenbaum never, ever cursed, and the impact of this word coming from his lips was enormous.

"Of course everyone covered my tracks," the chief continued. "Every doctor kills someone in his career, whether he knows it or not. Well, I thought I was immune, above all that. And then it happened to me. It will happen to you."

"I just made this horrible mistake," Dean whispered, his voice cracking. "A thirty year old woman presented with ..."

"Consider yourself lucky, she's going to live. Don't look so surprised, I know everything that goes on here. Dean, my job here is threefold. To run the place, you know, nuts and bolts crap, making sure the schedule is filled, credentials are up to date, things like that. Second, to provide the best medicine possible to whoever rolls through our doors, be they bank presidents or bank robbers. And finally, and this may be the most important thing of all, to develop a cadre of premiere physicians, men and women, who are going to make an impact on this world.

"It's not easy with the budget cuts, the new regulations, and the turf battles with other departments. There are people in this building, there are politicians, and there are people in the media who hate us and would just love to bring us all down. It's a constant battle out there, you have no idea.

"What you're doing could adversely affect everything. At your present pace you are definitely going to trigger a sentinel event, the worst thing possible. There would be an avalanche of investigators, bad publicity, and maybe even the Department of Health. I've worked too hard to let you screw things up. Not to mention the fact that it could ruin you, Dean. You're going to be one of the good ones."

"Can we get to the point?" Dean asked. He was starting to feel very tired.

"Yes, let's get to the point. I'm going to insist that you take some time off, effective immediately. From my calculations you're owed at least nine weeks vacation. As of right now you are off for the next two of them. You can take all nine for all I care—your goal is to rest and re-charge. And if I hear that you are moonlighting during this period, I will terminate your contract.

"When you return to work, two, three, four weeks from now, you are not ever to work more than forty eight hours in any seven day period. Are there any questions?"

Dean sat there, exhausted. He felt as if he weighed a million pounds and realized that he couldn't go back to the ER now even if he tried.

"No questions. So, if you'll excuse me," he said, slowly rising from his chair. "I think I'll sign out to Doctor Finkel. Thanks for not firing me."

"That option wasn't even on my radar screen. Good luck, Dean."

As he stood up, one of Dean's teardrops rolled off his nose and splattered on Tannenbaum's desk. The elderly physician had by now resumed looking into his large book and pretended not to notice.

chapter 27

Julie stretched lazily in her chair, noting with satisfaction how the men checked out her movements from the corners of their eyes. On this particular day the ER was extraordinarily, almost eerily, slow, and most of the staff was relaxing in the break room, sipping on coffee. It came in three strengths, regular, samurai and caveman. Today's brew was decidedly strong, pure caveman.

I'm going to the cafeteria," she finally announced. "Anyone want something?"

"Not me, I'm out of here in an hour," Ehler said. "We're having pot roast."

"I'd like some peanuts," Carol said. She was watching the men watch Julie, thinking about how hopeless they were.

"What did you say, you'd like some *penis?*" an intern leered. He was standing by a counter, writing up an admission.

"Peanuts, with a '*t*,'" Carol clipped. "You got a problem with that, Prince Little Meat?"

The intern's head seemed to snap back. He returned to his chart with pained casualness, his face a brilliant red, ignoring the chuckles and snickers from all sides.

"Never fuck with an ER nurse unless she wants you to," Finkel whispered to no one in particular. He and Carol exchanged glances. "And I think that calls for another cup of caveman."

"Well, ta ta, I'm off," Julie said. She got up and walked away, amused as always as she sensed the men following the sway of her small but very rounded hips.

"Doctor Finkel?"

"Yes, Harry." Finkel put down his puzzle and peered at the student, who he had been proctoring for the past several weeks. Finkel's role of teacher had heavily imprinted on the younger doctor, who now followed him everywhere, at one point even to the bathroom. Indeed, Finkel had lately been referring to him as 'my little duckling.'

"With pseudo-hypoparathyrodism , what's the response of urinary cyclic AMP to administered parathyroid hormone?"

"How the hell should I know, Harry?" he replied wearily.

The student blinked. "Sorry, Doctor Finkel, I didn't mean to bother you."

"What ever are you talking about. All right, let's see if we can figure this one out. You know, Harry, you're supposed to forget this stuff the day after your boards."

"Well, I have a nineteen year old male with a neck mass, low serum calcium and low phosphorus …"

"What, you have a patient with something other than jungle crud? A real medical case? I thought the guards were under orders to filter out humans. This is major. Carol, call in the media."

"Endocrine sure brings back memories," Ehler said. "I did a rotation in it, about a million years ago."

"Internal medicine is my first love," Finkel said, putting down his puzzle and leaning forward, a distant look about him. "The condition you are describing, Harry, known as PHP, is hereditary, and presents like clinical hypoparathyrodism, but the hormones just can't kick in on the cellular level, and the bones thin out. And yes, Harry, there is a normal urinary cyclic AMP response to exogenous hormone."

He looked around, beaming.

"I remember it," he said triumphantly. "In fifteen years I've never seen a case, but damn, I still remember it!"

Ehler leaned forward and addressed the student.

"Doctor Finkel answered your question, now you answer ours," he said. "In pseudo-pseudo hypoparathyroidism, what are the calcium, phosphorus and hormone levels, and what is the urinary cyclic AMP response to administered hormone this time."

Finkel and Ehler exchanged mischievous glances. Both had been internists before shifting into emergency medicine.

"I, I don't know," Harry stammered.

"Why don't you look it up," Ehler said. "By the way, what genetic syndrome is it associated with?"

"Sorry, I just don't ..."

"Albright's Hereditary Osteodystrophy. You've got to read up on this, man. Selectively forgetting is one thing, never knowing it is another. And you have to know this stuff cold for the boards. Remember, you're on loan from internal medicine."

"Sorry."

At that moment Dean walked into the room and sat down. It had been two days since his minor disaster in the ER and his subsequent meeting with the chief. Secrets being impossible to keep in this smallest of communities, everyone had a rough idea of what had transpired.

He looked around the smiled at them.

"Well, don't you look nice and mellow," Ehler carefully said, sipping some coffee.

"Yeah, what's wrong, Dean? You don't look crushed by overwhelming burden," Finkel said. "Is everything okay?"

"More than okay. I'm on vacation."

"Good for you," Finkel said. "I think I'll try one myself someday. By the way, how did things go with the field boss?"

"I'll give you the details later, but basically he cut back on my hours. Now it's my turn, Fink. How did it go with the, uh, you know, that lady ..."

"It never happened. Forget it. She's fine, by the way."

"It's forgotten. Now all I have to do is figure out where to go for a month. It's scary, all this time off. I didn't know what I'm really like anymore."

"Personally, I'd be afraid to find out. I might be a rotten person," Finkel said.

"Fink, you don't have to go away to find out—just ask," Carol said. She was applying nail polish, and kept her eyes on her hand. "Dean, where do you want to go?"

"Some place very remote, very far away. I want out of this crazy world."

"How about a beautiful beach resort, with warm water, frozen pina coladas and great food?" a resident asked.

"Too civilized. I'm thinking of backpacking. I might even sign up for a tour of the Amazon rainforest."

"God, a rain forest," Ehler breathed. "The absolute center of the world. Complete ecosystems, brimming with life and energy. Did you know that until recently rain forests comprised twenty percent of all land mass?"

"You don't say," Finkel said, sardonically. "Pray continue."

"Of course it's almost gone now," Ehler continued. "But I hear it's beautiful. I'd do it if I were you, Dean. I'd see it before it disappears."

"Just keep one thing in mind, Dean," Finkel said. "Some of those tribes down there are cannibals. One of their delicacies are maggot-laden brains. They eat the body right away but let the open head, well, ripen on the ground. When it is crawling with little goodies, they lightly sauté it. That's the truth."

"Thank you, Doctor Finkel, for preserving my diet," Carol said. "I just decided to shop through lunch."

"I'm just being honest with the man. When you get down to it, you can't go much higher in life than lying on some manicured beach and having a servant bring you drinks. Beside, why depress yourself, you see enough of human madness around here."

"It's not depressing," Ehler said. "Maybe we can turn things around …"

"No one's turning anything around," Finkel said. "First of all, there are too many people on this planet, like ten times too many. Of course they're going to use up the empty spaces, it's just common sense. And second, there's my theory about elephant leaves."

"What's that," Ehler asked.

"People in mud huts don't like wiping their asses with them, regardless of what you may think. They want scented toilet paper, tiled bathrooms, four bedrooms, and a heated garage—well, maybe not a heated garage in the jungle."

"It's good to see that your cynicism extends beyond medicine," Carol said, blowing gently on her fingers.

"Hey, poverty sucks. You know it, I know it, and now they know it," Finkel continued. "You can't stop poor people from trying to be rich. For better or for worse, everyone wants to be just like us. And it's a one way street—aside from an occasional college student or some wacko security guard no one ever tries to become more like them. And even the college kids come back, for all their talk. No, we preached modernism to the Indians, and they bought it big time. You fantasize they're happy rubbing dirt on their faces and drinking donkey milk, but they'll stop doing it the first chance they get. Just try taking their televisions away. You may want to save the Amazon but they don't. Hey, we wiped out our wilderness, why won't they? And why can't they?"

"So there are too many people, huh?" Carol asked. "You're a doctor. You keep them alive for a living. Explain that for me."

"Don't do as I do, do as I say. Besides, I need the money."

"Fink, you are so weird," Carol said. "It's a good thing you're cute."

"In other words, that crazy guy with the book had a good point after all," Harry said. "Get rid of the people, and you'll save the ..."

"Stop, stop, stop, now," Ehler insisted. "Don't get this started up again."

"He was a very crazy guy, and we'll leave it at that," Carol agreed, holding her hands up in front of her for inspection.

"Well, he can't be that crazy, he's still walking around," the intern replied, not looking up from his chart. "He was surrounded by a bunch of people, they looked like bodyguards. They treated him like a VIP or something."

"Who? Connigan?" Dean asked, leaning forward. "Where was this?"

"By one of the shelters. I passed it in a cab the other day. I guess the police didn't think the book was real. But that was some great story."

"I'm sure they already questioned him," Ehler added carefully. "See, Dean, it's over."

"Something is wrong," Dean said. "This guy is dangerous. You know, I found out he once worked on some microbiology project for the government."

"So what, he had to work somewhere," Ehler said. The phone on the table rang and he answered it. Then he stood up, making a face. "They want me in Room One. Fever and a rash. Another 'fever and a rash.' What's going on here?"

"I called Connigan's university," Dean continued. "He taught for a while, then was recruited by the military. He didn't last too long there, but they couldn't give any details."

"You mean he was too unstable to work for the government?" Finkel asked. "Now I'm getting nervous."

"This really bothers me, him walking around," Dean said. "You can make all sorts of poisons from the totally legal, easily obtainable chemicals. Bob, Dan, come with me to the security office. I want to talk personally to Officer Brandt."

"Come on, man, I've got work to do," Ehler protested.

"It'll seem more legitimate if the three of us go there to express our concerns."

"I don't have any concerns," Finkel said, slurping his coffee.

"Please, do it for me," Dean implored.

Finkel looked at Ehler, who shrugged and looked away.

"All right, we'll come along but this has got to be fast," Finkel said. " It won't stay slow forever. Harry, pick up a chart and cure someone."

The medical student bolted to attention.

"Alone? Thank you, Doctor Finkel, thank you. Uh, excuse me, can I speak with you?"

Finkel looked at Harry.

"What exactly do I do?" the student whispered.

"Grab a chart and practice what you learned. It's actually quite easy. When in doubt, order a test to stall for time—with luck you can punt the case into the next shift. Anyway, give erythromycin to all the men, and sulfa to all the women. And if you do kill someone, write it up so that someone else gets blamed. That's the secret of good documentation. Now, if you'll all excuse me, I'm off to save the world."

chapter 28

The three doctors strolled through the ER before heading for the Security Office, as Finkel insisted on making sure things were stable before he left. Dean walked by the familiar surroundings almost wistfully, the sights and sounds quickening his pulse. There were restrained psyche patients, screaming children, patients with lacerations, burns and broken bones; the range of pathology in this room was enormous.

"Nothing that won't wait," Finkel murmured, looking around. "Let's go."

Dean felt much more relaxed with Finkel beside him. His friend had treated the Connigan incident with cynical amusement; he knew, however, that others in the department already lost respect for him. For all his quirkiness, Finkel was highly respected and well known throughout the hospital. Here was a solid ally.

They passed a stretcher that had been left in the hallway. Patients in this section were for the most part admitted, and were waiting for either a bed upstairs or for transport.

Dean glanced down and squinted. One patient lay very still, a surgical mask draped around his neck. It always angered Dean to see potentially contagious patients left alone in public areas. Invariably these people would rip off their masks and place everyone at risk, exactly as this man had done.

He stared at the man, at his scars and tattoos. Something here looked familiar.

"I swear I know him," he said to Finkel, who was also staring.

They both recognized him at once.

"It's the Four Million Dollar Man," they said together. Four Million, as everyone called him, had literally earned his nickname. To support his drug habit over the years he had spent just about that sum of money, and it was obvious that his income came from neither the stock market nor digging ditches. Four Million was everyone's worst nightmare—a vicious, incorrigible, one-man crime wave.

"You could drive a freight train down those tracks," Finkel snorted, looking at the man's forearms with a mixture of admiration and revulsion. "He's injected shit into his body at least fifteen thousand times, and he is still walking and talking. Me, if I get so much as a splinter, I almost die. I tell you, these shpos are superhuman."

"Well, something sure caught up with him this time around," Ehler said. "He looks comatose."

"Positively angelic," Finkel said. "Come on, let's go."

"When I was a senior resident, Four Million was on my service, with endocarditis," Dean recalled. "One night he killed the patient lying next to him because the man was snoring too loud. He shoved paper down the man's throat and then went to bed. The only witness was some guy in DT's, you know, completely unreliable. They couldn't file any charges, but everyone knew what happened. Four Million even used to joke about it. He'd say, 'I told you I wanted a private room.' Nice guy, huh?"

"Like I said, angelic," Finkel repeated. "One of the founding fathers of that Death Master gang, I hear. This is a great day, he looks like he's finally circling the drain. He's got that last roundup look, don't you think?"

"Oh, damn, look at his skin."

Dean pointed to a pale rash that gently covered the man. The more they looked, the more obvious it became. Instinctively holding his breath, Dean leaned forward for a closer look.

Four Million opened his eyes.

Dean, only inches away, started badly, as if someone had just shouted 'boo!' He tried to move away, but the patient grabbed him by the arms and squeezed. Dean's eyes bulged in pain and surprise—he was shocked at the man's strength.

As quickly as it began, it ended. Four Million's hands fell limply back to their sides, his weakened muscles drained of their last reserves. He looked weakly at the doctor.

"He sure greets old friends in a funny way," Finkel said nervously.

"That really hurt," Dean said, wincing. "God only knows what he was like in his prime. I do hope he's not contagious"

"Wait, he's saying something," Ehler said, staring at the man.

Dean moved closer again, this time cautiously. The dying man was moving his lips, attempting to make sounds. His eyes resembled flickering candles.

"Doctor did this, your doctor," Four Million finally whispered.

"*My* doctor? What are you talking about," Dean hissed, his hair standing on end.

"Doctor X."

Dean turned and looked wildly at Finkel.

"Did you hear that," he shouted.

"Say that again," Finkel demanded, poking the man in the ribs. "Oh shit, he's crashing. Somebody call a code!"

A dietary aide was standing nearby. He ran over to a phone, pushed a button and spoke rapidly into it. Almost immediately the code alert roared over the wall speakers. Within seconds, seemingly from out of nowhere, the hallway was flooded with personnel. They surrounded the stretcher.

"He blamed Doctor X for this," Dean said excitedly. "You heard him, Bob. He said Doctor X was one of 'my doctors.' That must mean I know him or something."

"Well, whoever or whatever Doctor X is, my hat's off to him," Ehler said. "He's done what the justice system has been unable to do for years. This guy was bad."

They saw a surgical resident gloving up, holding a blue-wrapped cutdown tray between his legs as he did. They knew what was coming up—he was going to crack Four Million's chest and perform open cardiac massage.

"Disgusting," Ehler said with annoyance. "He's doing it right here in the hallway. Blood's going to get everywhere, and it's beyond high risk, not to mention worthless in a non-trauma case. You do know why he's doing this, he's showing off to Julie."

"Everyone's been showing off to Julie," Finkel said dryly. "I'm surprised people haven't been whipping out their dicks when they walk by her lately."

The narrow hallway was now swollen with people. Everyone seemed to be speaking at once. The three ER doctors let themselves be nudged out of the way.

"Well, if Four Million wasn't dead before, he'll be dead soon," Dean said. "That open chest technique is nothing but showboating. Let's go. Doctor X just notched another one."

They eased their way down the hall.

"So this was a premeditated hit," Ehler said, shaking his head. "You're going over the top, Dean. For years these people shared for same needles, booze and sex partners. They're lucky they lasted this long. Why must there be some evil conspiracy behind everything?"

"It all began after I found the book," Dean said. "That Connigan guy practically spelled out what happened to these street people, and one of them actually knew Doctor X."

Ehler interrupted him. "Hold it a minute. Hey, everyone, listen up! Use extreme body fluid precautions with his patient ..."

"Don't worry, Ehler, I won't kiss him," the surgeon quipped, hovering over the pulseless man. "If your little ER had more space we'd be playing this game in a room. Now, if you'll excuse me ..."

"Hey, fuck you and fuck your manners!" Finkel snapped. The resident looked at him, locked eyes with him for a few seconds, and lowered his eyes. The hallway quieted. Finkel glowered at the residents, and spat on the floor. He turned to his friends. "Come on, guys, it's calming down. Let's see what the police have to say. Let's put this crap to rest, once and for all."

chapter 29

After carefully washing their hand in a hallway sink, they snaked through a maze of corridors and approached the Security Office. This was the administrative section of the building and they were the only physicians there; there was no longer any hospital feel to the place. When they entered the Security Section—emerging into a large office with windows that looked out onto a busy side street—the atmosphere was that of pure police station.

In reality, that was the truth, this large public hospital being one of several that had a small but dedicated police office, which worked in conjunction with its security staff, most of whom were retired from the force. The room was filled with heavy-chested men with rolled up sleeves. Dean imagined they were detectives. Several uniformed police officers lounged nearby, sitting on folding chairs, sipping coffee. In a corner sat correction officers and sheriffs, waiting ꞏꞏꞏꞏ for their prisoners to receive their medical treatment and then take them back to jail.

Cautiously, they walked up to a desk, where a middle-aged detective with a crew cut sat, reading a magazine. Dean had never been here before, and felt slightly disoriented. He found the suspicious stares of the policemen disconcerting; strangely, he began to feel paranoid for no reason at all.

"What's up, Doc?" the detective asked, not looking up.

"Is Lieutenant Brandt available?" Dean asked, unable to take his eyes off of the man's shiny handgun, packed neatly away in its shoulder holster.

The detective looked as if he was going to ask why. Then he shrugged with boredom and turned around.

"Vic! Visitors."

Within seconds Lieutenant Brandt walked out of a side room and approached them. He was a huge man of about sixty, overweight but still obviously powerful. It had been rumored that he more than once had been involved in violent incidents, and had been transferred to this remote post in a last ditch effort to keep him out of further trouble. Through his physique had grown somewhat buttery, his facial features remained rock-hard, and his eyes cold and hostile. Dean couldn't help but feel fear in the man's presence.

"Can I help you?" Brandt said.

The room became quiet, and all of the officers turned to look at the doctors, who shifted uneasily at all the attention.

"Can I see you alone?" Dean asked uneasily.

"No, you can see me here," Brandt replied. "I got no secrets. Do you?"

"Okay, here goes. About three or four weeks ago Dr. Tannenbaum gave you a small book titled *The Words of Doctor X*. I was wondering what the disposition of the case might be."

"I don't know what you're talking about, Doc."

"The conspiracy book," Dean said, flustered. "The book by John Connigan."

"I don't know nothing about a book."

"The book about destroying the world. It details this incredible plot ..."

"Doc, I got work to do."

Dean heard contemptuous laughter around him.

"You've never heard of Doctor X, then?" he asked.

"What is he, some medical detergent? No, wait, a doctor from outer space. That's it, boys. A doctor from Mars."

Brandt looked around him, delighted at his own joke. He and several men began laughing loudly.

"I was under the distinct impression that Dr. Tannenbaum gave you a book. He said he was even going to call you at home."

"Like hell he would. I don't give my number to any of you. If you can't find me, it's because I don't want you to find me. Now, is that all?"

"He's just asking a civil question," Ehler said. "There's no reason to act so snippy."

Brandt glared at the doctor, who shifted uneasily.

"I know you. Is it Dr. Ehler?" he asked.

"Yes, I spoke to you a while ago about the chef in the French restaurant."

Brandt's eyes squinted.

"Now I remember. The guy who jerked off in the cream sauce. Yeah. You screwed me on that one. I fell for that crap of yours. We sent a team out to that guy's restaurant. We even taped him. You know what happened? He didn't, we got cited by some state agency and Central reamed my ass. I've had it with you guys. Now, is there anything else?"

With that, Brandt wheeled around and walked back into his office.

Dean stood there dumbfounded. He wasn't used to being talked to like that, and his powerlessness had an unsettling effect. He turned around to leave.

"Doctor, excuse me."

A nearby officer spoke to them. The words had the ring of an order. The three doctors looked at him, feeling as if they had been pulled over for a traffic violation.

"What's this about a patient's book in your possession?"

The detective was small and thin, but his eyes had a malevolent gleam in them. He smiled coldly at them. Alarms went off in Dean's mind. Careful, they warned, he's a bully.

He decided to act stupid. Let them laugh at me, he thought, don't get caught up in their games.

"Well, it's like this. The book states that aliens are transforming themselves into microwaves and beaming themselves onto Earth. They're hiding out in all these, you know, microwave ovens. Soon, when the time is right, they'll enter the brains of all those who turn on the oven and take control of the owner's body."

"And, uh, you believe this?"

"I don't know what to believe anymore."

The detective rolled his eyes around for all to see.

"Doc," he said loudly and slowly, to make sure everyone was watching. "I think you've been sticking your finger up too many assholes."

The entire room erupted into harsh laughter.

"I knew you wouldn't understand," Dean said.

"Oh, I understand, all right," the detective said. "Go back to your junkies, Doc."

Murmuring apologies, Dean shuffled out of the room followed by Finkel and Ehler. As the door closed they heard catcalls and hooting, followed by general laughter.

chapter 30

"That was ugly," Ehler said when they were safely away, headed back to the ER. "I can't believe we are on the same side as those ... look at this."

They were back in the hallway where they had seen Four Million. They approached the stretcher, lifted a blood soaked sheet, and stared at his gutted body. It eerily resembled that of a slaughtered deer. They looked into his chest cavity disapprovingly. A few feet away Gloria slowly mopped the floor; for a moment it looked to Dean as if she had been crying.

"What a mess," Ehler said. "I'm writing these people up. There's blood all over the place. Doesn't this stuff just tick you off?"

"I shocked and appalled," Finkel replied flatly. "I'm actually more ticked off about those cops. To think that I give them sick notes. What do you think, Dean?"

"I'm not worried about the cops, I'm worried about Tannenbaum. He lied to me."

"Tannenbaum?" Finkel asked. "The man who spends half his free time on soup lines feeding the homeless? You think he's behind this stuff?"

"It might be a cover, I don't know. But I believe more than ever now that somehow he's involved. I want to speak to him now."

"Sorry, Sherlock, but he's leaving for a conference," Finkel said. "He'll be back next week. Dean, life's too short to worry about this junk. This guy here was a creep."

Dean paused, deep in thought. Suddenly the idea hit him.

"Of course this guy's a creep, all these guys are creeps," Dean said, his voice rising. "That's the beauty of this plot. Four Million was just an experiment, a human guinea pig that no one will miss. I mean, who cares if a Death Master dies?"

Gloria stared at him coldly, threw her mop down, and walked away. They paid her no mind.

"It's up to us to stop the plot," Dean continued ."We don't have much time."

Finkel looked at him. "We? Ehler, say something, talk to him."

Ehler cleared his throat but didn't take his eyes off of the corpse.

"The premise is that since humans are destroying the world, why not destroy them first and prevent it," he said evenly, choosing his words carefully. "On the surface, it appears to follow a cold, but valid logic. Mankind is a dangerous pathogen, and the treatment is simply to kill it."

"Exactly," Dean said excitedly. "That's what I've ..."

"But it's the logic of evil, cruel, heartless evil. It's inhuman. Luckily, this plot thing is unrealistic. It's just too much for one man, or even one group, to pull off. And it is inconceivable to believe—no, it is impossible to believe—that Dr. Tannenbaum is involved. He's a normal person, Dean, like you and me. I've been to his house, and I met his family. As for this Connigan, he sounds like an end-stage psyche patient. Maybe he formulated a plan, and maybe he wrote it down. So what. I just don't believe it exists in real life. The scariest thing, Dean, by far and away, is that you are falling for this stuff. You're acting as if you almost want it to be true. Are things really that bad?"

Dean smiled at his friend and sighed. He felt a little foolish.

"What do you suggest, Dan?"

"Take a nice, long vacation, and recharge your batteries," Ehler said kindly. "The world will still be here when you return. By the way, these have not been fun conversations. I'm married, and I have three beautiful kids. Even speculating about ..."

At that moment Ehler's beeper went off.

"Trauma protocol, Emergency Room," it barked.

"Gotta go," Ehler said. "Dean, speak to me before you leave."

With that he turned and walked down the hallway, breaking into a trot halfway down.

Finkel looked at Dean and smiled.

"Personally, I'm rooting for the computers and cell phones. Screw the outdoors, too many bugs," he said, turning to leave. "I'm going to help out on the trauma. Let's meet tonight at Biggie's for some drinks, okay? The overall perspective of everything improves dramatically after two martinis, assuming they're extra dry, of course."

"Of course," Dean answered distantly.

"I'll see you there about eight."

Finkel walked away. Dean stood alone in the hall, leaning slightly against the lonely stretcher, his fingers absently drumming a beat on one of Four Million's legs as he swayed gently, deep in thought.

Stay cool, he thought. Get out of this place and go far, far away. Lie on a hot beach for hours. Let your biggest decision be whether or not to move into the shade. Forget about medicine and sickness and death. Forget about conspiracies. Forget about that marriage. God, I want to get away from everything.

He closed his eyes and let waves of fantasy wash over him. I want to go to the end of the world, he thought. I want to go to the end of the world. The end of the world.

He stood very still, breathing lightly.

"Hi, Doc."

Dean started violently. He jerked his head around, and saw a short man and a somewhat taller woman. He had no idea how long they had been there. At first he was very confused, but within seconds he recognized the man, a friendly street person he had treated several times.

"Hello, Toot."

"How you doing, Doc, it's been a while. This here is my friend Frenchie. Hey, is this guy dead or something?"

Toot prodded the body and shook his head sadly. Frenchie stared at the lumpy sheet with alarm. She was almost as tall as Dean, with a honeyed complexion and wavy, medium length hair. Underneath her clean but simple jeans and sweatshirt he sensed a full, well proportioned body.

One of her hands had been resting on Four Million's splayed open chest, separated only by a sheet. She recoiled as if shocked with electricity. Her eyes rolled backwards and her knees began to fold.

Dean had seen this happen a hundred times before. Quickly, he stepped forward and caught the woman as she slumped over. She crumpled into him, her head crashing into his face, stunning him for a second. Her breasts pushed into his chest. Dean struggled with the sensations of physical pain, sexual arousal and his professional need to care for someone in distress.

"Come on, you'll be all right," he said soothingly to her, not exactly sure where his motives were coming from. He held onto her tightly and started escorting her to a nearby chair. Toot ignored them, and lifted the sheet to stare at the body.

Suddenly Frenchie straightened and became alert.

"I'm okay," she said, turning to him. Dean looked into her eyes and felt he was about to start floating. Try as he could, he could only see deep, soft, blackness, which seemed to go on forever. I could get lost in her eyes, he thought. I could find eternity and the secret of life by just looking at her.

He stopped drifting and shook himself back into a professional bearing. After having held her gently, for perhaps a second too long, hoping she didn't notice, he let go. She stood up, holding on to the wall for support. Then she smiled at him, and the band in his chest grew even tighter.

"Thank you," she said shyly.

"You're very welcome."

"I know this guy," Toot said, still peering at the body. "He's like all the others."

"What are you talking about," Dean asked, the hair on his head rising.

Toot seemed frightened, and this was unusual for him. He was one of Dean's favorite patients, dating back from his residency days, and he still sought Dean out for all sorts of problems. He'd typically study the posted doctors' coded schedules—Toot and Bob McElvoy were the only patients to whom Dean had ever given his ID number, so they could find out when Dean would be working. He was a most unusual man, having been born into a primitive tribe deep in the Amazonian rain forest.

Named Tuti, he left as a teenager after his people's habitat was converted into grazing land,, his tribe melting into the surrounding shantytowns. After wandering for years, doing all types of work, he had wound up deep in this city, in this neighborhood, and here for the last few years he stayed, mastering the language and the ways of the street. He remained unique, however, nonviolent yet self-sufficient, warm and cheerful, yet distant. He lent the image of a visitor from space mingling with the local inhabitants. Dean was quite taken with him and looked forward to their meetings.

"He's like rest of them," Toot said, not taking his eyes off the corpse. "They all have this skin thing, and then they get real sick. That's why we were looking for you."

"You've been looking for me?" Dean asked incredulously.

"Yeah, something's happening. My friends are starting to die. Just like Four Million here, not that he was a friend. But something's going on. Five more just got sick this morning at the plantation."

"Where?"

"It's what we call our hangout."

"Tell your friends to come into the hospital."

"They're afraid. You know, they'd rather keep a low profile."

"They shouldn't worry. There are confidentiality rules. I just want to help them. Toot, it's vital that we make contact …"

"They won't go. You've got to come with me. Please."

Dean's mind raced. Could this be the connection, he wondered, could this be Connigan's testing ground? If nothing else, he might help stop an epidemic from breaking out.

He looked at Frenchie, who was leaning against a wall. She had been staring at him, and when he turned to her she became embarrassed. Dean thought her very enchanting. Her lips look like honey, he said to himself, and her skin reminds me of a summer sunset.

He heard himself saying, "Listen, Toot, I'll make a house call. One time only. When I get there, if I think a trip to the hospital can help them, you let me call an ambulance. Is that a deal?"

"You got it, Doc. Deal."

Dean felt strangely proud that this street person had personally cho-sen him for such a personal and important mission. Several of his col-leagues would have undoubtedly laughed Toot out of the ER, and several more would have called in the police to have him questioned. But Dean felt nothing but gratitude at having been selected. I'll just have to start my vacation tomorrow, he thought.

"Toot, I've got to go home and change, and also to get some equip-ment. Give me the address and I'll meet you there. Wait a minute, am I going to get killed if I go to this place by myself?"

"Don't worry, we'll go with you. You'll be safe. Go home, do your thing, and then come back here. We'll wait by the ambulance entrance. I got friends upstairs to visit, anyway."

Dean felt slightly uneasy, coordinating plans with someone who was both a patient and a notorious street person. He scrupulously main-tained the doctor-patient role in all his dealings, believing this to be the best and most proper way. He stole a quick look at Frenchie. Although he was certain he would never touch her again, he hoped he would never be her doctor, just so he could go on looking. Then he put on his most serious face and faced Toot.

"I'll be back in less than an hour. Wait for me at the ambulance entrance. If you're not there, then I'll know you weren't serious. And the deal sticks. I call for an ambulance the moment I decide it's necessary, okay?"

"We'll be there, Doc."

Dean remembered nothing of his trip home. Deep in thought, he kept picturing the events of recent days. When he entered his apart-ment he looked around nervously. It looked the same, quiet and some-what unkempt, nothing apparently amiss.

He stared at his closet, no longer sure what to think. He had by now convinced himself that it was he who had re-arranged it, perhaps in his sleep—recently he had started taking a sleeping pill notorious for causing sometimes comical, sometimes bizarre, sleepwalking be-havior, especially after a few drinks. Now, again, he was filled with un-certainty.

The possibility of a deliberate, conspiracy-driven epidemic chilled him. It started out almost like a glorious game, he thought, a diversion from my drab life, an escapist fantasy run wild. It wasn't meant to be this real. I was going to cure my boredom, not the world, and then go off on a nice, long vacation.

He walked over to a mirror by his dresser and leaned forward, looking deeply into his eyes. If there really is a conspiracy, he said to himself, moving his lips silently, it's going to get very personal very soon—I just may die, and very soon, considering that I touched two victims.

We need a plan, he thought. I'll examine Toot's friends, make sure this is on the level, call an ambulance, call the police, tell them everything and give them my copy of the book, this time right into their hands. An hour from now this case goes public.

He decided to change his clothes. What *does* one wear when saving the world, he wondered, half smiling. He selected khaki shorts, sneakers and a loose fitting cotton pullover. The informal safari look, why not, he thought. Now, bring on the bad guys.

Sitting on the edge of his bed, tying his laces, he thought of the virus. God, if it was real ... The suffering would be unspeakable. Imagine the plague's last days, the mass hysteria and fear. Cities burning, electric and water service gone, impassible roads, violent mobs.

Connigan had calculated an astonishingly high kill rate. Then, factor in the very young and very old survivors dying within weeks. At least another half slowly starve or die from lack of medicine. Without the even the basics of civilization, medical skills, or even common-sense survival techniques, the world as we know it just *shuts down* ...

He stood up and walked back to the mirror. "The bottom line is that within two years the world reverts to the Stone Age," he said aloud, looking into his eyes. "Most survivors will eek out a miserable existence and die miserable deaths. Everything we've worked for over the past thousands of years will vanish, practically overnight."

He started to leave and then paused. I should tell someone what I'm doing.

He walked to the phone and dialed the ER. Finkel wasn't there, his shift apparently over. He called Finkel's home and left a message. For good measure he left a message on Ehler's phone as well. Not satisfied talking to machines, he took a small piece of paper from his wallet and dialed again. A sleepy voice answered.

"Hello?" Helen said.

"It's me, Dean. I'm sorry I woke you."

"It's okay," she said, suddenly alert. "Where are you?"

"I'm home, but I'm going out. I wanted to tell you."

"Tell me what? Dean, are you okay?"

"Listen, I can't talk long. I'm going off with Toot, he's a patient of mine, one of my regulars. He's sort of a street person, I don't know how else to describe him. We're going to a place called the Plantation. He says there are sick people with symptoms like the ones we've been seeing lately."

"Dean, this is very dangerous …"

"I'm going to break this case wide open. Helen, I knew it, this Doctor X thing is for real. I don't care if you or anyone else thinks I'm crazy, I am going to find out what's going on. There's more at stake here than you can possibly imagine."

"Dean, this is not a good idea."

"No one's going to kill me. I've known Toot over fifteen years …"

"Never mind. Dean, if this is true, and I'm not saying it is, then it's bigger than you are. Call the cops if you want, but don't be a hero."

"Ma'am, I'm just doing my job," he joked, imagining himself the town sheriff going to a showdown.

"Let me come with you!"

The fantasy of he and Helen marching into the unknown to save the world was delightful. Hopefully, I'd get to knock out some bad buys, stop the epidemic and still get to sweep her into my arms, he thought. Then we'd go into the sunset, me and my sweet Helen, the woman with the sad eyes. I'd try so hard to make them twinkle …

"No, I've got to do this alone," he heard himself saying. "I promised Toot that it would be just me. He's pretty trustworthy. Hell, I saved his life at least …"

"Dean, please. Listen, I'm coming right over."

"Good-bye," he whispered. "Come to Biggie's tonight, eight-ish.

I'll regale you with how I saved the planet. And maybe you and I can have a talk, or something."

He gently cradled the phone into its receiver and padded to the door. This saving the world is rough stuff, he thought with a smile. As he closed and locked the door, he heard his telephone ringing. Turning, he trotted down his hallway and into the stairway. He flew down the steps, taking four or five at a time, swinging around the banister at each floor to increase his momentum. It was a habit he had developed as an intern, to allow him to run to codes faster. Somehow, he perceived himself to be in a rush. Within seconds he had reached the bottom.

chapter 31

Julie lay on the large bed, covered only with a soft satin sheet. She shyly looked up at Finkel, who stood over her, and absently licked her lips. Finkel smiled and gently knelt down on the bed, still not touching her. Julie opened her mouth slightly, breathing softly. She nodded to him, and with the barest of motions parted her legs … .

"Dr. Finkel?"

"What?" Finkel blurted out, almost in pain at having had his reverie so quickly shattered. He had been suturing a jagged leg laceration. The man, a house painter, had slid down a ladder when a rung cracked, a nail sticking out of the wood splaying his leg wide open. It was nice case to relax with, not particularly difficult but extremely time consuming. Aside from occasionally asking "how're you doing up there?" or "does this hurt?" Finkel was alone with his thoughts. Here in the minor trauma room, with the door closed, he was as distant from the main ER as he could be.

"Dr. Finkel? Are you okay?" Harry asked"

"What in God's name do you want."

"Dr. Miller called, he said it was important. I thought you had gone."

"Damn it, I was here all the time. Did he leave a message?"

"No, he said he would try you at home."

"That's just great."

"Can I watch?"

Finkel sadly nodded his head. His fantasy session with Julie would have to wait.

"Sure. Maybe I'll even let you assist."

"Oh, gee, thanks."

"Oh, gee, you're welcome. Do you want to learn how to suture?"

"Definitely."

Harry walked over and reached for a suture holder and needle.

"Harry, do you think you might want to put on some gloves, first?"

"Oh, yeah, sorry."

Finkel waited patiently while the student clumsily pulled a pair on. Was I ever really like him, he wondered in amazement as Harry battled to stick his fingers in their proper slots. At one point four fingers entered the thumb hole, at another all fingers entered their proper hole but the glove was on backwards. Finkel watched patiently, hoping against hope that Harry would die.

When Harry had won his war against the gloves, Finkel motioned him to lean over. He pointed inside the gaping wound.

"Listen, the most important thing is the need to maintain the sterile environment," he said. "You can perform the best closure in the world, but if you're sloppy, you'll get an abscess, and that can be worse than the actual laceration. You hear me?"

"Yeah. What are we looking at here?"

"It's a great anatomy lesson," Finkel said in hushed tones. "This particular area is split wide open, you can see everything. Look at this."

Harry leaned over even further. Finkel inserted gloved fingers from each hand and separated tissue for Harry to see.

"I could have given this to Ortho, but this cut is a beauty. Now, here we can actually make out the tibial plateau. If you just follow this imaginary line you'll see the head of the gastrocnemius tendon ..."

Harry had been peering earnestly into the ravine-like opening. As he shifted to get a better look, the sidearm of his glasses slipped off his ear and fell directly into the exposed area, nearly sinking out of view.

Finkel looked at him in horror.

"Why don't you just take a shit in there while you're at it!" he rasped.

"Dr. Finkel, if you had any idea how sorry I am …"

"Get it out."

"I don't know how it happened."

"Get it out!"

Harry reached in and fumbled with the sidearm. He pulled but it had snagged on something. Panicking, he gave a violent yank, and the plastic piece broke free. Suddenly, as if an angry volcano had been disturbed, the wound started filling up rapidly with blood, as a freshly ripped artery pumped its contents into the surrounding spaces.

"You hit a pumper," Finkel snapped.

At that moment the sidearm of the intern's glasses fell off again, falling back in the pool of blood. Instantly, Finkel fished it out and handed it over. He looked at Harry with a mixture of fear and awe.

"How'd that happen," the student wondered, looking at his glasses. "Damn, the tiny screw came out, that's why it came apart. Dr. Finkel, I think the tiny metal screw is still in there."

They both looked down into the bloody opening. Its surface pulsed with each heartbeat. Each prayed in vain that the piece of metal would float to the top.

"Someone sent you on a mission to destroy me, didn't they," Finkel said hotly.

" I'm really sorry. I messed up, didn't I?"

"Let me put it this way. You've taken the most delicate part of this man's leg and turned it into a toilet bowl. You may also have avulsed the medial tibial artery. Finally, there's a foreign body somewhere at the bottom of this mess. That pretty much summarizes the case."

"What are you going to do?"

"Harry, I think it's time to get some help. Put pressure on the wound."

Finkel removed his gloves and gown, keeping his eyes on the student, who was dutifully pressing the entire area with clean gauze. Because Harry looked so contrite, Finkel softened, deciding to ease up on him.

"Harry, do you like the ER?"

"I love it. Actually, I was thinking of going into the field."

"You're kidding," Finkel said warily. "What's your main reason?"

"Well, I never told anyone, but I really enjoy telling people their loved one is dead or dying. Also, I like making disaster announcements."

Finkel stared at him.

"I can't believe you just said that. Harry, just press the wound. I have to find an orthpod."

Finkel stormed out of the trauma room, shaking his head. Ignoring everyone else, he walked out of the ER and into the staff lounge, looking around him. To his great relief, a friend of his was sitting in front of the television.

"Oz, thank God you're on today."

"Fink, how's it going," the man said in a Southern accent. He was tall and blond, wearing paper scrubs, booties and a surgical cap. The two shook hands.

"I got a problem," Finkel said, sitting across from him.

Quickly, Finkel summarized what happened. When he was done his friend laughed and clapped him on the shoulder.

"It'll be a pleasure," he said. "Hey, you've scratched my back, now I'll scratch yours."

He was referring to Finkel's expertise with difficult cases, as well as his willingness to send injured patients home, with appointments for the next day. This spared the orthopedists from having to come in, which they were required to do if so requested. When Finkel was on, they all knew they wouldn't be bothered by minor problems.

They left the lounge and returned to the ER, Oz entering the trauma room to take over. Finkel walked to the Nursing Station and sat down, making plans on how to avoid Harry for the duration of his shift.

Carol walked over.

"What's up? You look upset."

"I was up that famous waterway without a paddle a few minutes ago," he answered. "Who needs Doctor X? I can kill all the people I want just with Harry at my side."

"Whatever are you talking about?" she asked.

"Never mind. By the way, you may not believe this, but Dean may actually be on to something."

"Don't tell me he converted you. You do know all that stuff is bogus."

"Well, the end of the world stuff, yeah, that's pretty obvious. But there is something brewing. A bunch of creeps all seem to be dying of the same thing. Who knows where they got it, but it could be intentional. I was there when Four Million died," Finkel replied. "He definitely said the words 'Doctor X.' And, it just so happens that Tannenbaum never gave the book to the cops. I was there when Dean spoke to them. Something's going on."

"Well, then you are going to be very happy, my darling super-agent. Administration wants the two of us to go right now to the Fourth Street Shelter. Infectious Disease asked Tannenbaum to send some people out there. Sort of like advanced triage."

"Maybe we could bring some advanced medical supplies with us, like soap."

"There's been an outbreak of food poisoning or something," Carol continued. "A few people have died, and three more are on respirators at North Central. Someone mentioned botulism."

"Interesting," Finkel said. "Something tells me we've already gotten a few customers. There's been some strange pathology around this place lately."

"Apparently we did. Four Million was from that shelter."

"Even more interesting," Finkel remarked. "But botulism? No way in a million years. The toxin spares the marrow, heart and brain. I can't remark on the other cases, but Four Million did not die from botulism. Interesting, indeed."

"Well, then I guess that's why Adminstration wanted you to go. You're the triple-boarded doc. And besides, Tannenbaum's leaving for a conference, Ehler's off, and Dean's on the shit list. I'm going to be your sidekick. This way I can also leave early and get in some shopping."

Finkel thought for a moment. Then he stood up, his face brightening.

"Come on, Sidekick, let's go. Anything to get away from Harry."

chapter 32

Finkel found the contrast between the ER and the outside world startling; the day was bright and sunny, the air practically festive. Beside him Carol fidgeted. She had changed out of her customary scrubs, and instead wore a light cotton sweater and a short plaid skirt. She winked at him.

"Nice day, ain't it?" she asked.

"Yeah, very. I usually don't notice the weather. Some of Dean's sensitivity must finally be wearing off on me."

"Don't worry, you're still the crudest person I've ever met."

"Now, now, you'll make me blush. Hey, let's take our time and go by bus, okay? I can't really say I want to go to that place. It's nicknamed the Ferocious Fourth. Even sociopaths avoid it. Maybe it will blow up or be condemned by the time we arrive."

"Fine with me. We'll just say we couldn't get a cab."

They walked over to the bus stop, on the corner of the busy street. Finkel looked at Carol and smiled.

"Damn, you look cute. You look positively female."

"You once called me a junkyard dog dressed in scrubs."

"That was actually a compliment."

"Actually, I took it as such. Here comes the bus."

The midday bus was fairly empty. They moved to the back and selected a pair of seats by the window. The bus rumbled along.

Finkel couldn't help but notice how warm Carol's thigh felt alongside his and with the gentlest of motions nudged his leg even closer to hers. To his relief she didn't move. They sat in silence for a few minutes.

"That was some gunshot they brought in before, wasn't it?" Finkel asked lightly, looking out the window.

"Tell me about it, his guts were dripping onto the floor," Carol replied. "Why are men so sloppy when they commit suicide?"

"To get back at their mothers," Finkel answered.

"Once I almost killed myself slipping on some brains after some guy shot himself," Carol confided. "It was like ice skating in there. I almost went down. I broke my fall by reaching out, and do you know what I grabbed onto? The inside of the patient's skull. I almost died of embarrassment."

They both laughed. Finkel looked at the window, chuckling.

"Hey, Fink, what's with that druggie security guard? I swear I saw him following us," Carol said.

"Who, Mr. Natural? Why would he follow us?"

"I have no idea. But I swear ⬩ he was ⬛⬛⬛⬛⬛. He even walked out of the building right behind us."

"Carol, you've been hanging around Dean too long. Natural is harmless. He was probably looking for some stuff to cop. I'm sure the dealers know him well."

"Ooh, look at that woman with those babies," Carol said, changing the subject. "Oh, so precious."

"They're cute," Finkel agreed. "You like children?"

"Me? God yes. I don't even care if I get married anymore, I just want kids. What about you?"

"Yeah, if I could have done it over, I'd have had a bunch already. Creating life is the secret of life, as far as I can tell. Re-cycling homicidal maniacs in the ER sure isn't."

Carol stared out the window. She opened her mouth to say something, then closed it. After a while she looked at him.

"Yeah, I know," she mouthed silently.

Carol appeared to be sad. Finkel blinked—in front of him was not the toughest nurse he had ever seen, but a woman struggling with her feelings. When he had joined this ER, she already had a reputation as one of the wilder people, one not known to shy away from either fights or one-night stands. Whereas most people were intimidated by her, Finkel had always admired her, and half seriously considered her his ultimate woman.

"What's with you, what's the problem? You're all hot and sexy. You can have a million kids."

"Can I tell you something?" she asked, looking at him. "I mean, I know we've known each other for years. First, I may look okay, but I have trouble with men. Unless they're on top of me I can't seem to hold on to one. I don't think I'll ever find a man to have a million kids with."

"You, no boyfriends? You used to date every cop in the world."

"That's my point. Every cop. Fink, I've never even gone steady. There's something about me that just turns people off. It's me, it's my fault. I guess deep down I want people to go away and then I act on it.

"I could have had kids," she murmured, looking down. "But I'd rather not talk about it."

"If it's any consolation, I also stink at relationships," Finkel half-joked, trying to lighten the atmosphere. "I'm at my best with over-doses—we're on the same wavelength."

"And then there's that old clock inside of me, just ticking away," Carol continued, ignoring his effort to change the subject. "I'm thirty-nine, and menopause runs early in my family. There's no shining knight on my horizon. In fact, you're the only man who doesn't run in fear from me. So basically, I think I've had my little run for the roses. There'll be no kids, as much I as want them. But thanks for calling me hot and sexy."

"I think you're gorgeous."

"Fink, you think all women are gorgeous. You have the worst taste I've ever seen."

"I agree—you should have seen my ex-wife. Let me re-phrase that. Even factoring in my bad taste, I find you extremely attractive. Plus, you have great tits."

"They're plastic."

"You bought 'em, they're yours. Now listen, and this is hard because I suck at feelings. You're a nice person. Wow, I really do suck at this. Carol, you have a great personality. I have always enjoyed working with you … wait, I have always loved working with you. I just get energized being around you. There, I said it."

"Wait a minute," Carol said, squinting at him. "You just said all these good things. How come you never asked me out?"

"Well, you always seemed to be going out with someone. And also, I don't particularly do well with people I like. And finally, I was married for the first few years, remember? I'd come to work in a bad mood all the time."

"Yeah, I do remember. Why'd you marry her, anyway?"

"We were the perfect couple. She was nasty and I was vindictive. Momentum carried us to the altar. Boy, did she have a temper. Cold and crazy, I used to call her. We each prayed we could change each other."

Finkel stared out the window.

"My kingdom for a calm, friendly woman who loves to fuck," he said quietly, half to himself. He turned and smiled at Carol, who winked at him.

"You're nice and calm," he said, staring into her eyes, suddenly fascinated by their greenish-brown color. "Except of course when you get cranky. Then you can subdue a dirtball with the best of them."

"Thanks, but you're the champ when it comes to that. I still remember that drunken sailor, you know, the nasty one from the park. God, after you got through with him he didn't move a muscle."

"Oh boy. Carol, I have a little confession."

"What's that?"

"You know why he laid there so quietly? When no one was looking I sutured one of his ears to the mattress."

Carol looked him, her eyes and mouth wide open. Finkel stared back, nodding his head. Then they both broke out laughing, so loud that everyone on the bus turned to stare at them. They finished the ride in silence, each occasionally breaking into a giggle.

The bus pulled up to their stop. Reluctantly, as if they were breaking a kiss, they got up and walked to the exit door, each thinking about how much they had just enjoyed each other.

They moved through the narrow side street in silence, heading for the shelter. It was a few blocks away, and they were still in a well-to-do neighborhood, an area frequented by tourists, who seemed to be all around them. At one point Finkel turned around quizzically and scanned the crowds, not quite knowing what he was searching for. Seeing nothing, he frowned slightly and continued walking.

When they crossed a particularly difficult intersection, navigating around people and construction equipment surrounding one of the many potholes, Finkel took Carol's hand and led her through. When they got to the other side he didn't let go, his lungs and mind each holding their collective breaths. Carol squeezed his hand and moved closer, until her shoulder gently touched Finkel's chest; in a surprisingly natural motion he found himself putting his right arm around her. They continued walking. Finkel realized that he was smiling broadly.

Along the way they passed a large hotel, the Algonquin, known as one of the most beautiful places in the city. Its lavish rooms always seemed to be written about and pictured in Sunday magazine sections. They paused in front of the carpeted front entrance, watching the uniformed doorman open a succession of limousine doors for the many guests.

Finkel stole a look at Carol. I always knew she was crazy, he thought, but I never knew she was just as nice.

Carol winked at him..

"What you looking at, Doc?"

"You, I never realized how much I liked you."

She stared at the red carpet they were standing on, astonished at how happy she felt.

"Me? You like me?"

"Very much."

"I have wrinkles. Look, see? Right around my eyes ..."

"Oh, stop. I like everything about you."

"Then how come you're not trying to seduce me?"

"I don't know, I'm afraid that you'd say no."

Carol looked down again.

"I wouldn't."

Finkel looked into the hotel, and then turned to Carol.

"How about checking in for a few hours—or a few days."

Carol nodded. "Yeah, I'd love to. Fink, I have a confession, and you can back out now if you … listen, this wouldn't be pure, you know, sex for me. I've sort of liked you for a long time. We're like two peas in some strange pod. You know, sometimes I think about you all the time, sometimes so much it hurts. Then I'd try to change my shifts so I could avoid you. And then sometimes I switch just to be with you. I'm sorry if I'm acting weird … ."

He kissed her. She seemed to freeze for a moment, as if stunned, then wrapped herself around him. For what seemed like forever they stood and kissed in the hotel lobby entrance, oblivious to the oohs and ahs of the passerby, some of whom snapped their picture while they embraced.

"You, really, like me?" Carol asked again, looking at him, her heart pounding.

"You're the greatest thing since potato chips."

Carols smiled, biting her lip. Finkel's passion, and weakness, for potato chips, was legendary.

"Come on, let's check in," he said.

"Do you have any protection? This is the middle of my month."

He looked at her. He seemed serious now.

"Do you think I'd make good father material?"

"You? The best. You're handsome, smart, big. Yeah, you'd have great kids."

"Do you want to mate? I mean, like, for life?"

Carol winked at him.

"Yeah, sure," she said. "Who knows, you may be the one."

Finkel took her by the hand and they walked into the hotel lobby. She waited, silently praying that things would work out, while Finkel got them a room. As they walked to the elevator she looked at him.

"What about the shelter?" she asked.

"What shelter?"

"The one we're supposed to be going to? What are we going to say?"

"It's not going anywhere. We'll eventually get there. If worse comes to worse we can even fake things and say no one would speak to us. I'm good at faking stuff."

"Not at everything, I hope."

They entered the elevator. He kissed her.

"No, not at everything."

The doors closed.

chapter 33

Toot spat noisily on the pavement and wiped his mouth. His friend Godfrey, who had joined him, leaned against a wall, reading a day-old newspaper. They waited by the hospital's ambulance entrance. It was one of their favorite hangouts, usually quiet and peaceful, the surrounding parking lot being extraordinarily open and airy in the midst of the sometimes suffocating inner city. The area had the added bonus of being safe, and as long as they made no noise they were left alone.

"You think the Doc is gonna show?" Godfrey asked.

"He said he would," Toot replied, looking around. "He could have said no. Why would he lie?"

"Maybe he turned scared. You know, deep down, these doctors are really afraid of us. They act like big shots in the hospital, but once they leave they become regular people, and you know what we do to regular people."

"I'd hate to think that Doc is afraid of us," Toot said, frowning. "He's such a nice man."

"You're breaking my heart. If you want the truth, they scare me more than I scare them—their turf is bigger. Remember, they own the world. Damn, the Mets lost again."

"Anyway, I hope he gets here soon," Toot said." The guys are starting to look bad. They're gonna die, just like Rape and IceMan before that. Same rash, same everything. Listen, some of the guys think they were poisoned. They all ate cookies some strange guy gave them at the shelter. A big, fat guy, talking to himself."

"And of course they ate a crazy man's food," Godfrey said absently, studying the paper. "It makes you wonder who was crazier. Damn, fourth place. What is this world coming to?"

"That big guy was out of it," Toot continued. "Talking about giving everything back to the Indians, how he was going to kill all the machines. Some people, they looked like Indians themselves, came in and dragged him away. Some people said they even looked like me."

"Wild story. The boys at the plantation, they all have the same shit?"

"Yeah, looks like it. That's why I asked the doctor to come see them. Godfrey, why would someone try to poison them?"

Godfrey crumpled the paper in his large hands, his huge arm muscles rippling. Then, after a contented stretch, he looked down at his friend, who seemed tiny next to him.

"Toot, my man, there are billions of people in this world, and if only one person in a thousand is a maniac, then you still have millions of them running around.

"Look at the tunnel people in the subways," Godfrey continued. "Some haven't seen the sun in years. They just keep living down there, eating rats, digging even deeper. They hate everyone. Who knows, maybe the fat guy is one of them."

"In a way I wouldn't mind if he did give everything back to the Indians," Toot said, smiling. "That's me, I'm pure Yamomani."

"Yeah, your folks used to own the jungle down there, right?" Godfrey asked.

"No one owned anything. Everyone shared, with each other, with the animals. There was plenty of everything. It was like heaven, and it went on forever. So beautiful, man."

Godfrey lit a cigarette and stretched lazily. "Giving it all back wouldn't bother me, I got nothing to give. Never did, and never will. I used to dream about owning a house and some land, but now that I'm playing it fair, I don't have a chance, I'll never make it."

"We're in the same boat. In a way the fat guy made sense. But it ain't right to poison ... hey, here he is. Doc, over here!"

Dean cautiously approached them, regretting that he had agreed to meet them here. He was terrified that he would be noticed meeting these people, especially wearing street clothes. Ignoring the several nurses and aides taking a cigarette break in the area—he thanked his stars none of them recognized him—he walked up to the two men.

"Hello, Toot," he said, trying to sound like a doctor talking to a patient. "Well, let's go now."

"Doc, thanks for coming," Toot said, extending his hand, which Dean shook, while looking around nervously. "You got class and you got guts. I want you to meet my friend Godfrey. He's gonna be our protection while we do our thing."

Dean froze. Why do I need protection, he thought, where am I going. What is Toot's last name, for that matter. He could be on the most wanted list for all I know. And this giant friend of his, I wouldn't want to meet him in a dark …

"Don't worry, Doc, there's nothing to worry about," Godfrey said. "No one's gonna touch you, that's a promise. First, I gave my word to Toot. Second, I owe you. You saved my sister once. She was ripped up by some dogs."

Dean looked up at him, trying to remember his face. Normally, he forgot cases within an hour of discharge and often had trouble recalling any single thing he had done on any given day. Finkel called it pressing the ER doctor's delete button. Against all hope he went through his inventory of his most horrible trauma cases.

Suddenly he locked onto an image of a large man, cradling a sobbing teenage girl in his arms, standing in the middle of the ER on a winter night, both dripping with blood. He found out later that this man had personally charged into a pack of ferocious dogs that had set upon his sister. She had stumbled across their lair while taking a short cut through a lot on her way home. Fighting like a wild man, he had torn her loose, and then carried her through the frozen night into their midst. Dean remembered, as if it were yesterday, their blood pooling together on the floor, and the absolute quiet that befell the ER when their presence was finally noticed. He remembered the man's dignity as much as by his magnificent physique.

"Is your name Blake?" he asked hesitantly.

"That's me. Godfrey Blake."

"Yes, I do remember," Dean said, smiling. He eagerly shook hands with Godfrey. "How's your sister?"

"Doing great, you can barely see the scars. She's in the Air Force now. Stationed in Hawaii."

"I'm jealous, but I'm really glad to hear that. Say hello, for me, will you?"

Satisfied that he knew both men now, and that he had reinforced his role as a physician, he turned to Toot and nodded. The smaller man immediately started walking. Dean and Godfrey followed. They soon crossed the street, where Frenchie was sitting on a parked car, waiting for them. She nodded at Dean, the slightest of smiles on her lips. He smiled back, grateful to see her again. The small group turned a corner and walked halfway down the deserted street. Then they stopped, while Toot and Godfrey whispered plans to each other a few feet ahead.

"How are you feeling," Dean asked the woman. He again noticed how pretty she looked, and although she was wearing the same bulky gray sweatshirt, he sensed that her figure was stunning.

"Okay, I guess. I'm sorry I passed out on you, but it was creepy touching that, that body. I fainted because the shock slowed my pulse down, right?"

Dean stared at her, his eyes widening.

"Yes, it's called a vagal reaction. How did you know that?"

"I read it somewhere."

Dean smiled, impressed. They waited for Toot and Godfrey to finish their talk. Meanwhile, Dean studied the hospital, which loomed down the street. In the late afternoon sun, it looked shadowy and mournful, and it needed repair. He was surprised—he never realized how unattractive it looked from this angle. And it's funny, he thought, it doesn't even face the community it serves.

A cab raced into the parking lot. Before it came to a full stop, a door opened and a woman ran out. It looked like Helen, but he couldn't be sure. Before he could confirm it, the figure ran into the ambulance entrance and vanished.

Toot and Godfrey turned to them.

"Okay, let's go," Godfrey said. "Doc, you and Frenchie stay in the middle, keep cool, and everything will be just fine. Toot goes first, and I'll be the rear gunner. That's a joke, Doc, don't worry."

"Exactly where are we going?" Dean asked, trying to maintain an aura of control.

"It's where we hang out," Toot said. "You'd call it an abandoned building. But it's a decent place, and there's never any trouble. I don't really know the street address. Don't worry, you'll be okay. I promise you."

Dean nodded nervously, determined to be brave. He had last felt like this several years ago, while being strapped in for a roller coaster ride, the tallest and fastest in the world. As afraid as he was of heights, the fear had vanished the moment he was strapped in—at that point events were now out of his control and he decided to both accept and enjoy the ride. And he did. I survived it then and I'll survive it now, he thought. And it turned out that I enjoyed it. Who knows.

"Okay, let's go," he said.

The party of four began walking in single file across an empty lot. At its far end, was a street lined with abandoned houses. Directly in front of them, between two crumbling buildings, was an alley. It appeared dark and lonely, but peaceful at the same time; it almost beckoned him. Dean couldn't help but smile—his mother had warned him so many times about these very places. With Toot in the lead they advanced toward it. Dean turned around. In the distance he could barely make out the ambulance entrance. The woman who looked like Helen was standing there, looking around, as if searching. Before he could think or say anything the little party snaked into the alley and disappeared, and he hurried to catch up. He quickly looked behind him— the world had vanished from sight. Something's happening, he thought. Somehow, in some way, things won't ever be the same again.

Book Two

chapter 34

Helen stormed into the ER, looking around. Mr. Natural, who was leaning against a wall, waved at her. She ignored him, scanning the room. Ehler was on the phone, wearily, angrily, arguing a case, Julie by his side, holding a chart. Helen approached and opened her mouth, but he raised a hand.

"Look, he failed out-patient therapy. That may have been reasonable then, but he's back, he's worse, and he needs admission ... no, I won't switch his meds, he needs to come in, he's febrile and has a white count of eight-hundred."

Suddenly his eyes bulged in anger. Clearly the other doctor had hit a nerve.

"As a matter of fact, I am boarded, and this is my job. Don't ever talk to me like that again! Do I ..."

Ehler started violently as Helen pushed a button on the phone, disconnecting the call.

"What the hell! I was talking ..."

"Where's Dean," Helen demanded.

"How should I know," Ehler snapped angrily. "Who gave you the right to cut me ..."

"He left with some street people," Harry interjected. "They cut across the parking lot and went into an alley across the street. I was watching."

Ehler's eyes bored into the medical student, who looked away nervously.

"He's going to get killed," Helen said, shaking her head.

"Tell me what's going on, Helen, and it better be good," Ehler hissed. "And talk fast, my shift ended a half hour ago. I'm on my time now. What's going on."

Helen looked at him, her eyes burning.

"He's looking for Doctor X," she said.

"Doctor Ehler?" the ward clerk called out. "Doctor Clark just called back. He said he was disconnected. He said to admit the patient to his service."

"Screw Doctor Clark," Ehler said distantly. He shook his head sadly. "Things are spinning out of control. Finkel and Carol aren't coming back. They called and left a message. They're running off to get married. Just like that. Bob is scheduled to work the next three days and no one's around to cover his shifts. He's never done anything like this, and I've known him for ten years. All the nurses are freaking out because of Carol. And to top it off, you're telling me that Dean Miller has basically snapped. He's looking for a comic book character, accompanied by a bunch of street people. So, where on earth did he go?"

"I haven't a clue," Helen said. There was hint of anger in her voice.

"That's it, this Doctor X game is officially over," Ehler said, slamming his chart to the desk. "People are dying, people are quitting, and now people are disappearing. Dean's gone off on some oddball odyssey. For all I know, he's getting sick, and has some kind of altered mental status. If you will excuse me, I'm going to the police. And not that sociopath Brandt. I've got a friend at the midtown precinct."

"I'll go with you," Helen said. "A cab took me here, it's waiting outside. Two witnesses are better than one."

"Lead the way. I want to put this thing to bed once and for all. This insanity has got to end."

"Who's Doctor X?" Harry asked.

"Someone who wants to kill you in order to save the whales," Ehler said wearily. "I'm signing out to Molloy, and then I'm out of here. I can't stand being in this place one minute longer."

Ehler left the station. Helen watched him disappear. She shook her head angrily, her fingernails rapping the countertop. No one noticed the security guard quietly walking down the hall and around a corner.

Harry looked at Helen. She was often referred to as the 'mystery woman' of the department, never socializing, and practically living in the ER or the library. Although several years older than her fellow residents, and even some of the attendings, this did not explain her distance. Theories about her abounded, none provable.

"To save the whales, huh?" Harry said, intrigued. "What's the big deal about whales?"

"Because there are too many of us, and not enough of them," she replied absently. "The balance is gone, so these people have decided to restore it."

"How do you do that? Arm the whales?"

"No, kill the humans."

"That's sick."

"You asked. Maybe it's fitting that a doctor gets to be the one to do it."

"Why is it fitting?"

"Maybe we've caused most of the world's problems."

"Doctors?" Harry asked.

"I'm just rambling, Harry," Helen said with exasperation. "This thing with Dean has really gotten to me. The bottom line is that there are a lot of people alive today who simply should not be here. In other words, modern medicine is flooding the planet with rejects, all of whom reproduce a lot more than we do. It's not very natural, is it?"

"If it's not very natural, why did nature let us get to this point?" a voice boomed.

They spun around to see the tall, foreboding figure of Tannenbaum by the ambulance entrance. He stared at them coldly, his lips tight. They felt awkward and mute in his presence.

"We were just talking," Helen said hesitantly. "Shop talk between cases. I didn't mean anything bad by it."

"Your conversation is unprofessional and inappropriate, and I won't have it in my shop. You want to talk crap, go outside and do it."

Harry and Julie both froze with fear. They had never heard the distinguished chief talk like this. Helen stood still, looking at him.

"Has anyone seen Doctor Miller?" Tannenbaum asked icily, ignoring their shocked stares.

"What if we have?" Helen asked tensely.

"Then tell me. I want to talk to him."

"You're supposed to be at a conference," Helen said, her voice tightening..

Tannenbaum walked up to her. Helen stood her ground, looking directly at him.

"I don't have to tell you anything," he growled. "Where is he? Mess with me and you'll be out of this hospital so fast your head will spin."

"And question number two, why didn't you give Dean's book to the police," Helen continued. "That wasn't very nice, was it?"

"It's none of your business what I do!" Tannenbaum snapped. "Don't get involved with that book. Where is Miller?"

Helen looked squarely at him.

"I'm not going to tell you."

They stared malevolently at each other. Harry and Julie held their breath, stunned at the confrontation. The room seemed to grow quiet around them, as Helen and the chief stood facing each other defiantly. Suddenly Tannenbaum broke his gaze, the anger gone from his eyes. He looked around the room, deflated. Harry and Julie looked around the room embarrassed and exhilarated at the same time. Helen's eyes continued to burn into him; Tannenbaum actually seemed to squirm under their intensity.

"If anyone sees him, tell him to come to my office right away," he finally said. "It's very important."

With that, he self-consciously turned and walked stiffly into his office. When he was out of sight the staff exhaled with relief—the tension had been exhausting. They felt as if they had just witnessed a street fight.

"Dr. Carpenter, I never saw you so hot," the unit secretary said nervously. "But I admire you. He had no right to talk like that. What's going on in this place, I've never seen it like this."

"Yeah, congratulations," Harry said. "Although I hope you don't get in trouble. Doctor Finkel said the most important thing to learn down here is staying cool. He said losing your temper is like masturbating, it makes you feel good for five minutes."

"He had it coming," Helen whispered distantly, staring at Tannenbaum's door. "I hate him so much."

"Why would you possibly hate him?" the secretary asked with concern. "Just because of what he said?"

"One day he will walk in hell."

She looked at Helen, taken aback by her remark and by the twisted look on her face.

"Why?" she asked cautiously.

Helen whirled around and looked at the small group. Her eyes blazed with emotion. They stared at her uneasily.

"Once I had a son. You didn't know that, did you? My one and only child. I had an abruption during delivery, it almost killed me. When I woke up from anesthesia I had just gone through childbirth and an emergency hysterectomy.

"I didn't mind so much, he was gorgeous. He always smiled, never cried, slept through the night. Of course his father, that bastard, cut out. One night when my little boy was four, he had a sore throat—some croup, some drooling. What did I know, I was a nursing student back then. I took him to the ER. The doctor took a quick look down his throat, whipped out a prescription and sent us home. It took about two minutes, tops.

"Three hours later my son suffocated from acute epiglottitis. I remember holding him in my arms while we waited for the ambulance. Just as he went out, he looked at me, and mouthed the words, 'It's okay, mommy, I'm not mad.' And then, he died."

They looked at her, unable to speak, Harry shifted uneasily, painfully aware of how little he knew her.

"That ER doctor was none other than Tannenbaum," Helen said. "He doesn't remember me, but not one day has gone by that I haven't thought of him. And I swear ..."

She looked at them, her eyes wild, almost crazed. Julie and Harry both averted her gaze, suddenly afraid of her.

Ehler's replacement, Carl Molloy walked up, holding a chart. The entire staff was grateful to see the doctor, grateful for the respite.

"Hey, everyone, what's going on?" Molloy said. "You guys see a ghost?"

"Where's Ehler?" Julie asked.

"I give up, where's Ehler?"

"He went to the other side five minutes ago to sign out," Harry said. "You didn't see him?"

"Afraid not. It's, shall we say, 'dead' back there. The weather's too nice, only sick people are coming to the ER today."

"He should have been back by now. Doctor Carpenter, don't you think ..."

Harry's voice trailed off when he saw Helen. She remained motionless, her face contorted with anger, her eyes boiling. He turned away nervously.

Julie scowled and walked hurriedly away. Molloy looked at her, shrugged, and went off to see a new patient. Harry looked at him, his eyes pleading.

"Doctor, can I go in with you," he asked.

"Why not, come on," Molloy said casually. "You know how to sew?"

"Doctor Finkel taught me," Harry said hopefully. ""He had this big laceration ..."

"Good, you're gonna be my 'lac man.' Let's get going."

"See you later, Helen," Harry said quickly, eying her nervously. He and the senior doctor walked around a hallway corner.

Helen stood there alone, not moving, her eyes fixed on Tannenbaum's closed office door.

chapter 35

For Dean, walking through the long alley was as alien as walking on the moon. After several minutes in this silent maze, concrete walls towering on both sides, he had lost all touch with the outside world. It remotely reminded him of a trek years before through a desert ravine. It had started out as a small crack on the hard desert floor, then slowly widened and deepened as he walked, the walls slowly appearing as he very gradually descended—eventually they towered over him on each side, blotting out everything else. He was totally isolated at that point, and these images and feelings came back now. Even the sounds were similar—back then it was the crunching of his boots on the sand. Now, it was the sound of cracking bits of glass.

After recovering from the initial jolt of this lonely, almost tomblike path, he began to find the trip strangely pleasurable, as if he were a tourist in another world. Aside from his companions there was literally no sign of life, and no markers to place where he was. I could be anywhere, in any time, he thought to himself, as they snaked through the alleyway.

They finally emerged into some barren, unrecognizable street, which led to an empty park. Forming a loose group, they walked through an opening in a tall, chain link fence and walked inside. Dean felt relaxed and reassured after a few minutes, after realizing that Toot and the others had passed up numerous opportunities for perfect, unstoppable crimes. If they were going to do something they would have done it, he thought. He practically swaggered across an open grassy field, savoring a new sense of invincibility. Most people are afraid to even drive around here, he thought, and here I am, taking a leisurely stroll.

"Nice place, isn't it?" he whispered to Frenchie as they walked through desolate stretches with half-dead trees. "I didn't even know this park existed."

"It was dedicated in 1731," she said. "The English used to hunt foxes here. After the tenements came everyone sort of forgot about it. Some people picnic along the edges, but no one really goes deep into it. It's too dangerous."

"What do you mean, 'dangerous'?"

"It's okay, we're with Godfrey."

"I hope so," Dean said, looking around, mourning his short-lived sense of invulnerability.

They saw no one on their trip and finally reached the far end, exiting through another opening in the fence. The street they emerged onto was in a state of disrepair, with giant potholes and craters pocking the street, and abandoned buildings on both sides. Dean had heard of it only from the ambulance reports. He kept looking around, as if trying to see the hospital, to give himself some reference point on which to anchor. Distressingly, the seemingly huge institution had vanished from the horizon; it was as if it did not even exist.

Late afternoon was rapidly fading, a thick grayness descending from the sky, blanketing the world around them. They kept moving, walking along deserted streets, the ultimate paradox in the so-called inner city. One block was dominated by abandoned, boarded up stores, each in various states of decay. Aside from a few cats picking their way along the gutter, the only sign of life was a group of teenagers gathered around the shell of a car. Without knowing for sure, Dean assumed them to be a local gang.

Several of them held half empty wine bottles, and others were swaggering and playfully fighting with each other, but they fell silent as soon as the little party approached. As they filed by, Dean felt their menacing glares and knew what they were contemplating; he sensed several of them tensing as if to strike out. He began to tingle with fear, numbly realizing that he was helpless, weaker and slower than everyone around him, completely incapable of either running away or fighting back. He suddenly felt ridiculous in his shorts, white socks and sneakers, having branded himself as little more than a middle class animal of prey.

But they made no moves or sounds in his direction, instead nodding deferentially to Godfrey, who smiled and nodded back at them. Like a tour guide who had just gotten his little group through customs, he signaled gently with his hand, and they continued down the desolate street.

Dean was unsure how to act, never having been in this world. Though he worked nearby, his patients had always come to him, on his terms, trading their independence and often their pride in return for his knowledge and curative powers. Now he shockingly was out of place and totally at their mercy, his former role, if anything, a deadly liability here. He found this new reversal disorienting, and was embarrassed at the fragility of his long held assumptions of law and order—he survived now only through the good graces of his newly acquired bodyguard. Godfrey turned around, somehow seeming to sense his unease.

"Nice day for a walk, ain't it?" he asked. He looked at Dean and winked.

Dean quickened his pace, so that he could speak with Godfrey, who led the group. The powerfully built man that strode easily down the street, surveying all about him calmly.

"Did you know those guys?" Dean asked him.

"I know everyone around here."

"They looked like rough characters."

"I guess."

"I have a confession, Godfrey. I was nervous back there."

"That means you're normal. Those kids are mean. Some are gonna be Death Masters one day."

"That horrible gang?" Dean blurted out. He held his breath, horrified that he had offended his guide. I'm such a stupid ass, he thought.

Godfrey only smiled at him. Then he looked away, as if signaling that he wasn't in the mood for further conversation. Dutifully, Dean moved closer to Frenchie. The group continued walking.

After traveling down several more blocks, Toot made a slight whistling sound. The others stopped. He pointed to a large apartment house,
six stories high and completely boarded up. Part of the upper floors had
begun to crumble, and the entire area around the building had been
cordoned off with orange tape.

Silently Toot walked up to it. Prying open a large plank, he squeezed
himself inside, disappearing into the darkness. Godfrey and Frenchie
followed silently, and they too vanished. Dean was alone in the street.
He viewed the huge building with alarm; it seemed on the verge of
collapse. Fear seemed to bolt his feet to the ground. *I don't want to go in
there*, he thought nervously. *Why can't they bring the patients out to
me.*

He struggled with his indecision a few seconds more, until he saw
several rangy youths, all darkly clad, criss-crossing through an adjacent
lot, watching him all the while, as if stalking him. Calling for help would
be useless; his voice would never reach Godfrey, and he had not seen
any sign of the police since leaving the hospital. The youths came closer.
Suddenly the looming building seemed much friendlier; it practically
beckoned. Without further thought he ran across the street, tore open
the wood covering the empty doorway and plunged inside.

chapter 36

He found himself in a large lobby. It was shadowy gray inside, a trickle of the day's remaining light squeaking through various cracks in the walls and windows. The lobby was lined with surprisingly intact mosaic walls, each showing mythological scenes. For a moment Dean stared intently at them, captivated by their beauty, impressed all the more because this sight was so unexpected. Then he visibly started, realizing that the others were nowhere in sight. Anxiously, he looked around. With effort, he made out the outline of a large metal door, facing the rear of the lobby. He quickly walked up to it and pushed it open, hoping to reunite with his new friends.

He emerged into a small inner courtyard, lined on all sides by the building's towering walls. No doubt this area had once been quite elegant; now it seemed like the center of an urban tomb. Dean looked up and saw the darkening blue sky, squarely framed by the surrounding rooftop; it looked an eternity away.

Dean turned his gaze downward and was riveted by the bizarre scene before him. Six men, in two neat rows of three, lay on the ground. Three were already dead—it was obvious to his trained eye by their waxy skin color. The others were unconscious, most likely in shock, but still alive. A few feet away Toot and the others huddled nervously; now it was their turn to be frozen with fear.

Wordlessly, he walked over to the men on the ground. His sneakers made crackling sounds on the rubble. It occurred to him as he approached that these patients were no doubt contagious, and a warning voice in his brain told him not to touch them directly. Red alert, it said, big time pathology.

Cursing himself for not having brought gloves with him, he looked around for something, anything, to cover his hands with. Finally, in desperation, he ripped off a small piece of his shirt and wrapped it around his hands. Not that this is going to protect me much, he realized, just as long as it makes me feel better.

He knelt at their side and began to examine them. After taking each man's vital signs, he checked their eyes and ears, examined their skin, listened to their hearts and lungs, and palpated their necks and abdomens. When he had finished, he sat down in front of the men, on the cracked courtyard floor, stunned.

All of these men indeed had the same illness, each manifesting the now familiar rash, the same one he had seen in the ER. The thousands of small red dots that covered them indicated a drastically low level of platelets, the clotting agents of the blood. Each man had enlargement of his liver and spleen—one quick touch of the abdomen belied their massive size. All had an irregular pulse and were in mild heart failure. None even seemed dehydrated, indicating a rapid, ruthless disease.

"It's got to be viral," he said, looking at Toot. "Except for the stuff in the ER, it's not like anything I've ever seen before. I don't have the slightest idea how they caught it.

"One thing really bothers me. The men here seem to be at a nearly identical stage of this illness. Even these three who just died have the same skin temperature. Everything's within a few hours of each other. Normally some people are just coming down with something they just caught, others are in the middle of it and others are coming out of it. Whatever they have, they caught it at the same time. That's very unusual."

Toot and Godfrey looked at him blankly. Frenchie smiled at him, impressed.

"Doc, I don't know what you're talking about," Toot said finally. "But you're the boss. Tell us what to do."

Dean rose to his feet and faced them, unwrapping the cloth from his hand and throwing it in a corner, reminding himself to wash his hands vigorously as soon as possible, praying he hadn't been hopelessly exposed.

"I'm too late for them," he said, gesturing at the three bodies. "These others, they need to go to the hospital right now. As far as I can see, they have hours to live."

Godfrey looked at the sick men, his face a mixture of sadness and resignation.

"You know them?" Dean asked.

"Death Masters. A long time ago we used to run together. Damn, I never figured they'd die of sickness."

He bent over one of them and gently lifted an arm. Letting go, he watched it flop onto the ground. He turned and poked another man in the ribs. There was no response.

"Can't you do something?" he asked Dean, a pleading note in his voice.

Dean was about to respond when he looked up and saw an old man standing in the doorway from which they had entered. He was small and dark complexioned, with a face streaked with red paint and practically tattooed with wrinkles. One of his eyes was clearly sightless and had scarred completely white. Dean was stunned into silence at the incongruous image of what seemed to be an ancient Indian amid this urban wreckage.

"No one can help them," the old man said. He spoke with a slight accent, similar to Toot's, that Dean couldn't quite place.

Dean looked down at him, trying desperately to orient himself and maintain control of the situation. The last hour had been for him a trying time, a kaleidoscope of bizarre sights and sounds.

"What do you mean by that?" he said, trying to sound authoritative, "I'm a doctor."

The words sounded comical and practically devoid of meaning, slightly reverberating around the strange crypt-like courtyard. He looked around for support. Godfrey was looking around, his eyes darting everywhere. Toot was staring at the old man in a reverent trance, oblivious to all else. Dean turned to Frenchie, who looked at him nervously. She walked quickly over to his side. Then they both turned back to the old man.

"You can't help them," the man said. "They will all die. They are supposed to die."

"Are you a physician?" Dean asked, knowing the question was absurd.

The old man smiled gently.

"No? Then let one take care of them," Dean said with false bravado. Years of role playing, sometimes under the most adverse of circumstances, were paying off. "Toot, go call an ambulance."

Toot didn't move. He seemed to be paralyzed.

Slowly the old man walked up to Toot and touched his shoulder.

"It's good to see you, Tuti. I knew you would come back. Wait with your friend inside, in the big room. I want to speak with this man."

Toot nodded, and Godfrey shrugged. Without a glance back they exited through the door. Dean stared at Frenchie, who looked at him and shook her head wildly, indicating that she had no idea of what was going on.

The man approached them. Frenchie grabbed Dean's arm and squeezed it. Dean stood his ground, charged with his new role as protector. He and the man stared at each other, the dead and nearly dead all around them.

The man sat down carefully. He smiled at Dean and Frenchie, his face creasing in what seemed to be a thousand places, and beckoned them to join him.

"No one will hurt you," he said, sensing their fear. "Sit down. Both of you."

Very reluctantly, with a fatalistic air, Dean complied, followed a second later by Frenchie, who sat very close to him, her leg touching his.

"They'll be dead soon," the man said, gesturing at the sick men.

"You did this to them?" Dean asked warily.

"In a way. They are lucky now, their lives have not been wasted. Before, their lives were evil."

"They don't look very lucky to me," Frenchie said meekly.

"My dear, you are going to die, I am going to die, and they are going to die. It doesn't make any difference how long you live, only how you live, and for the first time, the lives of these men have great purpose."

"You like them being so sick?" Frenchie asked.

"Sometimes I feel sad. Many things make me sad. Your world makes me sad."

"Why does 'my world' make you sad," Dean asked.

"You would not understand."

"Try me."

"If you insist. Your world has destroyed everything in its path. It permits no life but its own. I swear that you people are from a distant star. Only that could explain why everything was in such harmony until you came along. In a thousand years you have undone a billion years of paradise."

"In the first place, I don't have any 'people,'" Dean said indignantly. "Secondly, I have not destroyed anything. I spend all my time making sick people better. And finally, what does this have to do with these men here?"

"They are warriors in the great struggle, and they make me proud," the old man said. He reached over to caress one of the dead man's feet, and then turned to Dean. "I have heard fine things about you. You are one of the good ones. Tuti shouldn't have brought you; you weren't supposed to see this. But it doesn't matter now. No one will ever find them, no one will even miss them. That is why we selected them."

Dean's mind reeled. He thought of the recent deaths at the hospital, and of the men lying on the ground here. Possibly this small man sitting in front of him was responsible; he certainly seemed to be taking credit for them all. So I stumbled right into the heart of it, he thought. I proved the conspiracy thing so much it's going to kill me.

He knew it was potentially dangerous, but he couldn't resist asking the question.

"Are you Doctor X?"

The old man's good eye seemed practically to blaze at the words. He looked at Dean, who with effort fought back the urge to cringe, although the gaze of this man practically made the back of his head burn. Dean closed his eyes until he felt its power wane. After a while he opened them a crack and looked at the old man, who was smiling.

"You do know a lot, don't you," the man said softly.

His mind swirling, with fear of confronting a murderer, with excitement at having solved a giant puzzle, and joy that he had been right after all, Dean didn't know what to say. It's real, he thought over and over, this whole thing has been for real. It was all on the level.

"You're the one?" he heard himself finally saying. "You are the mad scientist in the book?"

Frenchie looked at him nervously, shaking her head with the barest of motions. Quiet, she said with her eyes, don't blow any chance we have.

The old man smiled.

"My name is Juniactl. Some people like to call me Jungle Man."

Frenchie's eyes widened. She put a hand on her chest "I thought the stories about you were made up, like fairy tales. You're a real person?

"He's famous," she said to Dean. "People talk about Jungle Man. He's like the long lost king of some tribe. The last of them, or something. Word is it that he never goes out during the day, and, and that he won't look up at the sky until the day he returns to his land."

She looked at the old man.

"That right?" she asked.

Jungle Man smiled.

Dean tightened his lips, shaking his head. Great, this is just perfect, he thought. We're chatting with a mass killer who's part vampire. I broke every rule in the book by coming here. Unless I start acting a lot smarter, I'm a dead man. It might not be a bad idea to get the hell out of here.

Making rapid calculations, he decided to escape through a opening he had noticed in the wall to their left. He speculated that a window had once been there. Now all that remained was a thin piece of wood covering a hole.

Going back through the door would be useless, he reckoned, since this person undoubtedly had brought others with him who were likely to soon emerge from that very place. Violence was not an option, either, in part because of these presumed followers and partly because Dean couldn't bear to contemplate attacking this half-blind elder. He had never once been in a fight, and he knew he was incapable of hurting this man.

With one hand he rubbed his forehead, and with the other he touched Frenchie's leg, squeezing it several times, as if in code. She patted his arm twice, and he prayed it meant that she would go with him. Frenchie, I hope to God you're reading my mind, he said in absolute silence.

Jungle Man tapped him on the knee.

"You will both stay here, while I make ..."

"Now!" Dean screamed, leaping to his feet, pulling Frenchie up alongside him. They hurled themselves past the old man and raced towards the wall. Dean slammed his shoulder into the dry wood, which shattered with the blow. His momentum carried him through; in an instant he had disappeared. After a second's pause, Frenchie dove through the hole, and she too vanished.

Jungle Man had not moved. For a few moments he sat very still, listening to the crashing sounds in the building, which grew more and more faint. When all was still, he touched his ear, his knee, and then his opposite hand. There were scurrying sounds all around him, as his warriors obeyed his hand signals and began chasing their quarry.

chapter 37

They plunged ahead, staggering through the cavernous building, enveloped in a thin darkness. Navigating the long hallways was nearly impossible, the twilight providing only the faintest trace of a path. Dean kept thinking how poor their chances of escaping were. I'm sure these people know every square inch of this hideout, he thought.

They charged up creaking flights of stairs and ran through hallways, panting and wheezing with strain and fear. Frenchie stumbled on a step, and Dean picked her up; seconds later it was she who came to his rescue. This pattern repeated itself several times, as the two ran wildly through the darkness.

Finally, they reached a dead end—the stairwell at the opposite hallway had collapsed; it was impossible to get through. Dean imagined he heard footsteps. Impulsively, he opened a door they were running by and pulled Frenchie inside.

Almost immediately they crashed into the near wall. Putting out a hand he felt around, and realized at once that they had entered some type of small storage room. There were no windows and no way out. The sound of footsteps became louder. Quickly, quietly, he closed the door behind them. Drenched in sweat, not moving, they waited in absolute silence.

The sounds became louder. It seemed as if they were being chased by several people. Unthinkingly they grabbed each other and held on tightly. Padded footsteps sped by their door, as their hunters continued down the hall. Within seconds, all was silent again except for their deep breathing.

They were engulfed in complete blackness, clutching each other, afraid to move. The little room was warm but thankfully not oppressive. After a while, when it appeared that the immediate danger had passed, they relaxed, but didn't move their arms, or move away, only partly for security. In this tomblike hideout, devoid of all light, sound or reference to anything familiar, the only thing they had was each other.

Frenchie was the first to speak.

"I'm sorry they brought you here," she whispered. Dean was surprised at how sweet her breath was. "I had no idea, and I know Toot didn't either. I swear he loves you. You ought to hear the way he talks about you."

"I want to believe you. In a way I've always considered Toot a friend," Dean whispered back, trying to be cheerful. "But I would hate to see what he does to his enemies."

"I'm telling you, he didn't know. Godfrey didn't either."

"Godfrey, the protector. What the hell was with him?"

"Doctor ..."

"Dean. Call me Dean. I mean, we're about to get killed in a storage room. You can drop the formalities."

"Dean. Anyway, Godfrey has honor. Maybe it was seeing his friends dying like that. Maybe that Jungle Man just got to him."

"Jungle Man. Another class act. Where do all these people come from? I know I'm a boring, middle class person, but I never knew bad neighborhoods were so, well, bad."

"I'm sorry they brought you," Frenchie whispered again. "It was a terrible idea."

He continued to hold her, appreciating her softness, delighted that she didn't move away. It occurred to Dean that their bodies seemed a perfect fit. He felt her breasts against his chest and imagined he could stay like this forever. The recent horrors seemed remote and unreal in the blackness, and Dean gratefully welcomed their banishment from his thoughts. He fantasized that soon they would be able to sneak out and crawl to freedom.

To his shock and mortification, he realized he was getting aroused as he rubbed against Frenchie. Not now, you idiot, he screamed to himself. But the more he thought about it, the harder he became. Embarrassed, he tried to shift a little so as not to be discovered. To his great surprise Frenchie continued to cling to him, placing the side of her face on his shoulder.

"Men are all alike," she whispered, laughing quietly to herself.

"Sorry," Dean whispered back, not knowing what to say.

After a few seconds she lifted her head. Dean imagined her looking at him; in the thick darkness he could almost feel her eyes looking deep into his.

"Don't be sorry," she said. "And thanks for trying to help us, you risked everything by coming here."

She reached up and kissed him, finding his lips with a surprising ease. He held back for a moment, and then, as if intoxicated by her taste, kissed back hungrily. Frenchie responded in kind, holding him tightly and rubbing his back.

Their embrace seemed to take off and get a life of its own. They swayed together in the tiny room, each caught off guard by each other's passion. That grave danger that lay only a feet away, on the other side of a flimsy wooden door, made their desire even more urgent and more unreal. Dean's mind was spinning as he held Frenchie even closer. It's crazy. I'm being hunted down by a pack of killers, and I'm falling in love in some closet, he thought. Almost like dying in a gun battle after making love—the Fink would be proud of me. And he might be right. Somehow, I'm not as afraid of dying now.

And then all thoughts vanished as he lost himself completely in her kiss.

It seemed as if it could have gone on forever, had they not heard something down the hall. They reluctantly pulled apart and craned their heads in the direction of the sound, still clutching each other. Clearly, a door to door search was taking place, as each apartment on the floor was being entered. Muffled voices were heard; they appeared to be coming closer. Dean felt the fear coming back, but not as much as before.

Dean turned to Frenchie, his face inches from hers. He imagined he could see her.

"They'll be here soon. When they open this door, I'll rush them. You cut to the right. Maybe you can get out."

"I won't leave you," she whispered.

The sound of padded footsteps came closer.

"You have to," he said. "There's no use both of us being captured. Maybe I can distract them long enough for you to get away."

"I'm staying with you."

Dean felt her eyes staring into his. This is the strangest conversation I've ever had in my life, he thought, and I can't even see who I'm talking to.

"Frenchie, if they're going to kill me, they're going to kill me. We can't stop them, so you might as well save yourself. Bring the police here and tell them what we saw here."

"I'm not ..."

"Please, there's not much time, they're one door away. Who knows, maybe you'll even be able to rescue me."

"Okay, if you put it like that."

There was a scratching sound at their door. Dean closed his eyes, trying to brace himself for his attack. He loosened his grip on the woman.

"They're coming. Get ready."

There were sounds in front of their door. They seemed inches away.

"Frenchie, one quick question. Why did you come in the first place. I never asked."

"My brother was one of those Death Masters. He was one of the guys out there dying."

The doorknob creaked ever so slightly, and the door cracked open. His senses heightened in the absolute darkness, Dean knew that there was more than one person. Get ready, he thought, get ready.

The door slowly began to open.

"Run!" he screamed, crashing against the door, slamming it violently against what seemed to be several men. Frenchie ran past him as he charged into the group before him. He imagined himself a savage animal tearing into a group of startled prey, and two men were quickly knocked down with his wildly thrown punches. He was grabbed from behind but managed to break free. Rather than running away he plowed again into them, punching, kicking and shouting at the top of his lungs. Dimly, on the periphery of his thoughts, was a sense of satisfaction at his power and aggressiveness.

There were many of them and they came down from all angles. Finally he was grabbed around his knees and tackled to the ground. Several men jumped on top of him, crashing punches into his body and face. Still he struggled, oblivious to the pain, focused totally on battling on.

Finally his arms and legs were completely pinned and he was helpless. After a few seconds he dimly realized that they were no longer hitting him, and his will to fight seemed to soften. He lay on the ground, exhausted, his panting sounds filling the air along with those of his attackers. He briefly considered attempting to break free, but their hold on him seemed too secure, and with Frenchie gone—there was no sign of her in the darkness—it was hard maintaining his intensity. He had neither the desire nor the anger to fight on.

Surprisingly, the men around him did not punish him. They, too, seemed not to have the will to continue the violence. Rather, they dragged him to his feet and pulled a cloth sack over his head. To Dean, this seemed unnecessary in the near complete blackness of the hallway, and one of his eyes was nearly closed anyway from a blow. They prodded him into moving and led him down the hallway. After going several feet, they hoisted him on their shoulders. He felt them carrying him downstairs, comprehending nothing but the warm blood that seemed to be trickling out of both his nostrils and of how difficult breathing was becoming.

After going down what seemed several flights, judging from their repeated turns, they came to a halt. Dean's only thoughts were of his blood, which seemed to be drenching his face and neck. When they dumped him, roughly, on what seemed to be a soft dirt floor, he lay still for a second. Then, he slowly brought a bruised hand to the front of the sack and squeezed his nose in an effort to stop the bleeding. They beat the crap out of me, he thought, but they didn't kill me. What the hell is their game.

He heard a crunching sound on the dirt, as if someone was approaching. The silence around them seemed to deepen. He lay very still, his eyes wide open in the sack, seeing nothing, waiting. Instinctively, he curled up on the ground.

A bitter smell seeped through the burlap, stinging his already battered nose. Before he had any time to react at all he felt his arms jerked to his side and his head grabbed firmly. Part of the sack covering his head was lifted, and suddenly he felt a searing pain stab into the nape of his neck. He screamed in shock and outrage.

In seconds the burning ebbed, and his neck had a warm, numb sensation to it. The arms holding him released their iron grip and the sack was pulled off. Dean's first sensation was of the cool air on his sweaty face. In spite of himself he savored the feeling. Then, with a suddenness that surprised him, he unthinkingly jumped to his feet.

"What are you doing?" he said indignantly, not sure what he could or should do. Then he looked around him and his mouth gaped open in disbelief.

chapter 38

He was in a small torch-lit chamber surrounded by a group of twenty or so men who he could only describe as South American Indians. He had half-expected an urban street gang or wide-eyed cultists or even foreign agents in trench coats, but not this, and his first impression was almost one of amusement. That quickly passed when he noticed their long knives, and then he remembered his painful ribs and swollen nose, which still trickled blood. All the men were solemn, and they appeared so serious that after a few seconds Dean found himself accepting their presence. I've seen enough strange things today to last a lifetime, he thought, one more won't make much of a difference.

They eyed him with sullen hostility, as if they wanted, but weren't permitted, to harm him. That they could have killed him a hundred times over but did not emboldened him, and he stared back, noting that each had identical red streaks on his face, and eyes that burned with a blackness so deep they seemed to have no center.

There was a slight movement behind them, and without looking around they parted. Jungle Man walked into the room. He sat down wearily and beckoned Dean to join him.

"I tire so easily now," he said, looking up at the doctor.

Dean lowered himself to the ground, wincing in pain, knowing there was no choice. He had left all social power, all cultural leverage, on the street outside.

"What are you going to do to me?" he asked, trying to sound casual.

"Nothing," the old man said idly. He reached out to touch Dean's face. Dean winced nervously, but didn't resist. The man turned his face back and forth, examining his wounds. "You shouldn't have run away. Now look at you."

"What do you mean, 'Nothing.'"

"I mean nothing. You will stay here, in this room."

So this is some sort of prison, Dean thought, looking around at the barren concrete walls, which flickered coldly in the light of the torches tied onto posts in each corner.

"Look, if it's money you're after, I don't have any."

"No one wants your money," the old man said.

"Are all these guys from the jungle or something?" Dean asked looking at the men surrounding him.

"No, but will they be."

"What does this mean?"

The old man looked at him silently.

"Where am I?" Dean asked, trying to hide his growing desperation. "Can I ask questions?"

"Ask what you want," Jungle Man said. "You are in a special room, and you will wait here until the new day has begun."

"What new day? Please, if this illness is what I think it is, there won't be any new day. We'll all be dead."

Jungle Man smiled at his words, his face creasing again in what seemed to be a thousand places. He looked away, and all Dean saw was his white, sightless eye.

"If that is true, then I will die a happy man," the old man said. "I no longer thought that was possible."

"Do you know Doctor X?"

"Yes."

"And you know Connigan?"

"I know both of them."

"Then you must know that they're dangerous ..."

"No. It is you who are dangerous. We were told to capture you yesterday. You made it easy by coming here."

"Capture me?" Dean asked incredulously. "Who ... wait a minute. Does this Doctor X know me?"

"Yes."

As if a knife had stuck itself deep into his belly, Dean felt sick to his stomach. That this person was real was bad enough; that this person knew him was terrifying. He felt naked and manipulated.

"Who is he?" he asked in a quavering voice.

"Someone who likes you, apparently. That is why you were protected," Jungle Man said, indicating Dean's neck. Dean involuntarily touched the mark, which was staring to swell just a little. He remembered seeing similar burns in the past few days, but couldn't place where or on whom, having not paid them much attention. I believe him, he thought. God help me, but I believe him.

"Why was I 'protected.'"

"It is not for me to say. Probably you are a good person. I hope so."

"Who is this doctor?" Dean asked. "We must be very good friends."

"A gift from the gods. Someone who will restore harmony with the earth and sky, the one who will spare what is left."

"It's not right to do this, or even think about doing this. I read Connigan's book, so I know what you're talking about."

Jungle Man shifted on the ground and looked directly at Dean. His good eye blazed with intensity.

"I grew up in the forest, where sun or rain never touched the ground. Our ways were those of our ancestors, and we were at peace with the world. When I was a boy, the men from the cities came. We had never seen anyone outside those in our tribe, and from Tutu's group, who we traded with. We greeted the newcomers warmly, with gifts and food, with knowledge and stories about the forest.

"One day they informed us that they had claimed all our lands, which they described as 'wild' and that we now belonged to their government. We were declared savages, without rights or power. The few who resisted were shot, and not permitted burial.

"Our lands were cut down to grow coffee and spice, and we became slave workers on their new farms, living in tin huts. We, who had lived in the forests for untold years in peace and dignity.

"I saw five of my uncles die one day to settle a wager among the new masters, who had been drinking. They were arguing about how many men a bullet could travel through, so they lined up my grandfather and his brothers, all in a row. Five men fell to the ground, shot through the heart. My grandfather was the sixth man.

"The men laughed and exchanged money, and then walked away. What I remember most was the look on my uncles' faces just before the trigger was pulled. It was one of the deep sadness and, yes, fear. But it wasn't fear of dying, it was fear that their world, the one they had known and loved, no longer existed, that evil had triumphed over good.

"When my grandfather died I left my land, many years ago, on a bright sunny day. All that remained of my tribe was a pathetic band of broken people. My last act in my homeland was to hunt down and kill the men who had killed my uncles. I remember cutting out their hearts in anger, but the anger would not go away. All I could do was leave and never look back and somehow try to forget.

"It was beautiful on that final day, the air was so warm. I swore right there, as I was boarding a freighter that would take me far away, that I would never again look at the sun until, somehow, the invaders were conquered, and I could return and begin our ways again.

"These men around you come from many different places, but all have two things in common. First, every one here is a victim of your world. Yours has destroyed theirs. And second, and most important, they are all going home very soon."

Dean looked at the old man, speechless.

"In other words," Jungle Man said calmly, "now it is our turn."

"So it's your turn," Dean said, after a while, dabbing some blood from his nose onto his sleeve. "And everyone is going to die, except for a chosen few. May I ask, who are those lucky individuals?"

"Mostly the original peoples," Jungle Man said.

" 'Original peoples?' Something tells me that my family is not considered to be 'original.'"

"The few surviving tribes, scattered across the world," Jungle Man said impassively. "There aren't many left. They will be spared. A few from your society as well, but only a few."

"Why just a few," Dean blurted out angrily. "Are you afraid we might start kicking ass again ..."

He caught himself and held his breath, aware of how foolish his remark was, and how inflammatory it sounded. They could kill me in a second, he thought to himself. God, I'm a stupid idiot.

"I'm sorry for that," he said. "I'm tired, I'm in pain, and really upset by the things I've seen in this place."

None of the men seemed to mind, however, and Jungle Man actually smiled, his wrinkles deepening even more, shadows from them lining his face like black markers.

"I think you understand now," he said. "Your people enjoy ' kicking ass', it seems to be their true religion. They will die, they will all die."

"Who gives you the right to kill all these people?" Dean asked weakly.

"No one. No one gives out any rights. You killed us. Now we can kill you back. Why is it your right to use this world as you wish? Because you have submarines and spaceships, and we don't? We are simply taking back what you took, no more, no less. Like I said, it's our turn."

"Don't you have any idea how many innocents will die?" Dean asked. "Most people are good and honest. They didn't do anything. They love their kids. You just can't do this."

"My people lived in peace for thousands of years. We hurt no one. In the space of a century we disappeared from the face of the earth. We didn't do anything. And we loved our kids as well. Yes, I think we can do this."

"But it's just not fair," Dean nearly shouted. "Only a very small group did any of this. Why punish everyone?"

"Your civilization is large, and has many faces, good and bad. It is not possible to eliminate just one side. Everything has to be removed. Otherwise, the same situation arises, because the power, and the needs, of your world are still in effect."

"Do you have any idea of the suffering you will be causing," Dean asked helplessly, not knowing what else to say.

"It can't be helped," Jungle Man said, slowly standing up, wincing slightly from the pain in his creaking joints. "Anyway, a few days of illness is not suffering. Seeing your way of life desecrated, seeing your children grow up in a filthy shack, condemned to hopeless, joyless lives, that is suffering."

With effort, he straightened himself and stood erect. He made the slightest motion with his hands, and there was movement behind him. Suddenly, Frenchie was led into the room. One of her eyes was puffy and blackened. They pushed her next to Dean.

"You will wait here, the two of you," the old man told them. "In one week you will be allowed to leave. There is food, water and candles, and the toilet and sink in the side room work. Don't try to escape. You can't."

He and his men slowly filed out of the underground chamber. Jungle Man, who was the last to leave, turned to Dean as he closed the door.

"If you wanted to know, your living conditions here are better than those of half the people in the world."

The thick door clanged shut. They were alone.

chapter 39

Jungle Man and his followers made their way to the room where Toot and Godfrey were waiting. The two men, who had been lounging idly, stood up respectfully when he entered.

"As I said before, Tuti, it is good to see you," the old man said.

Toot beamed at him.

"You knew I would come back. I always come back."

"I know, our lives were meant to touch at many points. Though we are from different clans, our blood is the same. We have the same dreams."

Toot looked at Godfrey.

"Juniactl took me in when I wandered into this city. I was alone and very frightened. He raised me like a son, and I love him."

Jungle Man touched the younger man's arm tenderly, and then he looked at Godfrey.

"I hear you are a good man."

"I try," Godfrey said with a shrug.

"I want both of you to listen. I am going to scratch your necks and put some medicine on them. It will give you protection from the illness you saw. And then you may go. I want your word that you will not mention this place, or what you saw, to anyone. Can you do that?"

"I give you my word," Toot said without hesitation.

Jungle Man nodded. He had no doubt about Tuti, who he thought of as a son. Then he looked at Godfrey, the giant about whom he had heard so much. He knew that Godfrey once lived an evil life, and that he was a leader of the men in the courtyard. And that he had changed and become an honorable man, much loved by the people around him. To leave this bad group he had to endure many physical challenges, and the scars that marred his face he wore proudly, signifying to the world that he had been reborn.

"And you?" he asked Godfrey.

Godfrey put a hand to his mouth, and rubbed his lips, deep in thought.

"These men were once my friends."

"You must trust me that their lives are vastly better, now that they have not lived in vain. Please promise me. I will believe you, because I know that you are a truthful person."

"Where are Frenchie and the doctor?"

"They are well, and both have received the protective medicine. They will remain here for one week and then they will be released, unharmed. This is my promise to you. We won't hurt them. They are good people."

Godfrey turned to Toot, who nodded at him, as if to say, yes, what this man says is the truth, it is always the truth. He looked at Jungle Man and smiled.

"Who would I go to anyway? Okay, I promise. What I saw today will die with me."

"Good. Now lower your heads. You will be receiving the special protection."

In a moment it was done. Jungle Man looked at them.

"You will avoid all contacts with the authorities. You will keep out of sight and you will stay out of jail. We will find you when the time comes, and then you will understand everything. Our paths will cross again, and we will face the future together, under the bright sun. Do you understand?"

"Under the sun?" Toot asked incredulously. "With you?"

The old man smiled and nodded.

"Now go, both of you. I promise only one thing—good things will be happening very soon."

As Toot and Godfrey exited the room, each touching the burn on their necks, Jungle man sat down heavily. He had been looking for Toot and was glad to have seen him. But he had taken a very big chance sparing Godfrey and had broken his own orders about dealing with intruders. Indeed, two of the victims lying in the courtyard were homeless people who had wandered into the compound—they had been used for test models, as Mr. Natural had specified. But if Doctor X can choose to save a doctor, he thought, then I can spare my adopted son and his best friend. And yes, I will send his sister a dose, wrapped in some food. I will get her address.

   He felt the need to sleep and slowly arose. Signaling to his men, he walked out of the crumbling laundry room and went upstairs, for a quiet nap. The warriors melted into the building's deepest recesses.

chapter 40

The silence really is deafening, Dean thought in amazement, looking around the underground chamber. The cracked stone walls seemed to absorb the flickering candlelight; an overwhelming yellowy grayness surrounded them. The square shaped room was small, with fifteen foot walls, a low ceiling, with an alcove tucked in the far corner, presumably where the toilet and sink were. Aside from a large, dusty mattress which lay on the ground before them, and a squat table piled with candles and cans of food, the windowless room was bare.

This must have been some type of store room, he thought to himself. God only knows where we are. The passageways in these old places go on forever and interconnect with other basements. We could blocks away from where we started.

He paced the small room, trying to get a feel for it. The crunching sound his shoes made now seemed harsh and unpleasant, and he found himself taking them off so that he could walk barefoot. As if anything I did now made a difference, he thought.

"Are we trapped?" Frenchie asked, standing by the table. She had barely moved since they had been locked inside. Dean, who had been lost in thought, looked over at her and saw the fear in her eyes. A trickle of sweat was running down her face, glowing dully in the yellow light. He decided to lighten the mood.

"So, do you come here often?"

"Are we trapped?"

"Yeah, I guess we are," he said heavily, unable to force any humor.

"Are we going to die?"

"No, I think we are just going to stay trapped. We'll probably come out of this alive. If those people wanted us dead, we would have been dead long ago, it would have been easy. After all, there are bodies all over the place …"

He stopped, realizing that her brother was one of the victims in the courtyard.

"It's okay," she said sadly, reading his thoughts. "Maybe that old man is right, maybe he is better off. He was always so angry, and he did so many bad things. The law was going to catch up with him anyway."

"Anyway, I figure they'll let us out, I hope," Dean said, relieved that he hadn't mortally offended her. "Once they finish doing what they're doing. As for escaping, so far it doesn't look too hopeful. There aren't exactly any exit signs posted in this place."

"It's creepy down here. It's a cave."

"Yeah, like a cave. Something like my first apartment, only a lot more cheerful."

"You're something else," she said. "We're locked up in some dungeon, and you're making jokes."

"It's ones of my habits. I'm not sure if it's good or bad. When I get nervous or depressed I make stupid jokes. It got me through me for fourteen years of marriage and some pretty wild shifts in the hospital."

"You're married?" she asked quickly.

"I used to be. No more."

"Well then, joke all you want."

They both laughed, in spite of the situation. Then Frenchie's face turned serious.

"What's going on?" she asked.

"It's crazy. As far as I can tell some people want to release some bug, some germ, into the atmosphere. They want to destroy the modern world with an epidemic. It's a half-baked scheme."

"You mean they want to start another plague? Like the one in the Fourteenth Century?"

"I guess. You know about the Black Death?"

"I read about it," Frenchie answered. "It killed off a third of the world."

"Well, don't worry about this one," Dean said, trying to fake bravado. "I don't think they'll go very far. I don't think those guys could take over a restaurant, let alone the world."

"They're not trying to take it over," she said, biting her lip.

"Oh, they're just trying to kill everyone in it. A minor difference."

Frenchie started to cry. She stood by the table, shaking with emotion. Dean walked over to her.

"I can't believe this is happening she said," she said. "My brother's gone, I'm trapped, and a lot of people are going to die. My poor mother …"

Dean stared at the ground. I don't have one good thing to say to her, he thought. He had an overwhelming urge to touch her and comfort her, and he reached his hands out. She held his hands with hers—they fit perfectly, Dean thought—and moved a little closer.

"It's just not fair," she said wearily, shaking her head. "This life has been so crazy. I want a do-over. I want to wake up and be a little girl again, in my big bed, and have my future in front of me. And I'd say to myself, wow, that was a bad dream. The way it's been, God, every day has been like climbing a mountain."

Dean looked at her helplessly. She's a beautiful, intelligent, sensitive woman. A week ago we were probably passing each other on the street, not noticing each other. It's pathetic, it takes some onrushing apocalypse to meet someone like her. Maybe they're right, the world is crazy.

"You watch, things will be okay," he said. "Hey, are you hungry?"

Dean pointed to the food on the table.

"I don't know. I guess I could eat a little."

They let go over each other, and smiled. Then they both reached over to look at the food, and banged their heads together. Both jumped back in surprise and pain, each rubbing their head. Then, looking at each other, they began to laugh. Their laughter became wilder and louder, until it filled the entire room, until they were nearly doubled over, their eyes glistening with tears. Whenever they caught each other's eye, the harder they would laugh, at the horrors they had seen, at the macabre joke being played upon them, at their bodies' pains.

Finally, slowly, the laughter subsided, interrupted by an occasional giggle. Dean found himself touching her arms. So soft, he thought. He pulled her forward. To his amazement she didn't stiffen or pull back. She stood there and let him hold her. Holding his breath he pulled her close and hugged tightly, feeling her against his chest. She reached out and her arms encircled him. There was resignation all about her.

Dean wanted to say something romantic to her, something that would sweep her off her feet. He opened his mouth, but was unable to speak. The horror and the sadness that was all around overwhelmed him. Against all his self control, he found himself starting to cry. Frenchie looked up at him, her own face lined with tears, and then buried her face in his neck.

They stood there, holding each other tightly, rocked by emotions, each mourning, for stillborn dreams and for those that had died, for a world that used to be and for one that was never was. They swayed back and forth, yellow and orange light dancing all around them, hugging with all their might.

"I don't really know what's going on," Frenchie quietly whispered, knowing that Dean couldn't hear her. "But something is happening, I know that. These people are real, what they're doing is real. If I do have to die, please let me die with you, Dean. My last wish is that I can die with you in my arms."

chapter 41

The leader of the Death Masters squinted through his cigarette's curling smoke, lining up his shot.

"Four in the corner," Killer rumbled.

He sank it easily, grunting in satisfaction. The hulking shadows around the pool table nodded, and respectfully tapped their cues on the floor. The social club that was their headquarters was quiet, no one daring to create even the faintest noise. As always, when Killer took his games, the lights were turned down except for those over the table.

As Killer stalked the table, looking for his next shot, the wall phone rang. Quickly, one of his men ran over to answer it.

"Killer, it's for you," he said cautiously. "She says it's important."

The huge gang leader spat in disgust, annoyed greatly at having been disturbed. He walked to the wall phone, bumping two men out of the way. Neither said anything, each melting into the smoky darkness. Killer cradled the receiver.

"Yeah."

"Killer, I got to talk to you," the voice said.

"Gloria, I'm busy."

He was about to hang up, when the housekeeper shouted into the phone.

"I know who's killing your people!"

Killer's eyes bulged in surprise. Several of his men had gotten sick and died, and others had simply vanished. He'd heard reports of them being captured, but could confirm nothing. Inquiries on the street as to what was going on had been fruitless—the situation kept mysteriously deteriorating. That Gloria, a cousin working in the local hospital, should even know of such goings on was outrageous.

"What the hell you talking about," he demanded angrily.

"One of the doctors around here is using them for experiments," she said coyly. "He even wrote a book about it. He's been showing it off in the ER."

"Yeah? What doctor?"

"Someone named Dean Miller. He's been talking about this stuff non-stop. This book of his has plans for even more of us. Oh, and Killer, you should have seen Four Million, it would have made you cry. I mean, we grew up with him ..."

"Where's the doctor now?" Killer asked, his emotions boiling.

"Take care of him real good. He gave me trouble at work, he ac-cused me of stealing someone's ring."

Killer carefully wrote down the doctor's name and address on the wall. He hung up, and stared at the phone, his teeth clenched in anger. Suddenly he ripped it off the wall and threw it across the room. It smashed into the far wall, shattering into pieces. His men remained motionless.

"Diablo, come over here. I got a job for you."

Obediently, his lieutenant walked over, sidestepping the remnants of the telephone. He listened intently while the gang leader issued his instructions.

"And remember, do what you want, but bring him back alive," Killer concluded. "Take two of your best men, just don't mess up."

Minutes later three Death Masters, the toughest members of the area's most dangerous gang, stormed out of the club, heading for Dean's apartment house.

chapter 42

Mr. Natural poured tea for Connigan and Jungle Man, and then some for himself. They were seated around a small table in the headquarters' kitchen.

"Everything is ready," the guard said, blowing into his cup and taking little sips. "Amazingly, we're ready to go. We met our projected launch date. I mean, we'll release at the very hour we first said we would. Not bad, huh?"

"I could have used a little more time," Connigan mumbled. He stared into his tea, watching wisps of steam swirling on the liquid's surface.

"I wouldn't bring that up if I were you, John. That botch-up in the ER nearly …"

"Our success was meant to be," Jungle Man gently interrupted. "The gods are on our side. The hospital incident did not disturb me."

"Then you're a better man than me. I thought Connigan here really sank us. Listen, Doctor X wants you to summon your warriors. After the house is inactivated they are to drop from view."

The old man laughed softly. "They've been invisible from the beginning. They have no documents. There's no need to disappear, they never existed."

"How convenient," Mr. Natural said, mildly irritated at the old man's patronizing tone. "They are to assemble at our locations in the forest tonight to begin final preparations. They will remain by the cabin, guarding our supplies, but keeping the lowest possible profile. Understood?"

"I think we know how to melt in the woods," Jungle Man said.

"In three days everything will be complete," Connigan said, still looking into his tea. "The main components have already been linked. Remember, once the process starts, it cannot be reversed."

"That's the idea, now, isn't it?" Mr. Natural said, looking at the scientist.

"I guess so."

"We will do everything that has to be done," Jungle Man said, matter of factly. "For many years we have been praying for this. We will not fail. We can never thank Doctor X and the professor enough."

"The weather should be perfect, at least in this area," Mr. Natural said, hiding his pique at not having been mentioned. "When the survivors recover from the shock of being alone they will need all the help they can get. This warm spell, and summer being around the corner, should keep them alive."

"Thank goodness for that," Connigan mumbled.

The heavyset scientist suddenly stood up, his chair scraping the ground as he pushed it back.

"I have a headache," he said. I'm going to lie down."

With that he turned and walked to the door. Without looking back he left the kitchen. The two men at the table could hear his footsteps down the hall, which stopped at his room. Mr. Natural shook his head and then poured some honey in his tea.

"He is so strange," he muttered.

Jungle Man ignored the remark. As always he was astounded at how different from each other all three of them were. We're almost like an orange, he thought, appearing whole and complete on the outside, yet peel away the skin and we would fall apart at once. And here we are, part of a team, discussing the final details. It is our destiny come true.

Years before, the old man had wandered into a library, homesick, determined to look at pictures of his homeland in a travel book. The security guard happened to be seated at a long table, surrounded by books on the Amazon, looking at pictures of the rain forest. Jungle Man sat down beside him. They soon began talking.

"So you're from the center of the universe," Mr. Natural had told him, an impressed look in his eye.

"Perhaps you could say that," Jungle Man replied politely.

"It's disappearing at the rate of a mile a minute, doesn't it just kill you?" Mr. Natural asked.

"It hurts me, yes. Have you been there?"

"No, but I will one day."

After that initial conversation, they started meeting regularly at the library. One day Jungle Man was asked how important it was for him to return home. I would do anything to go back, he had answered. I do not want to end my life in this strange city. It was then that Mr. Natural introduced him to Doctor X, who was quietly forming a group to save the world.

So it happened that Jungle Man joined the small but earnest conspiracy, bringing with him more than twenty friends, men who had migrated from small, traditional villages across the world, men whose past had been destroyed and who had no future, men he had befriended and looked after. Men he could trust.

Very little progress occurred in the next few months of research and planning, and soon everyone was despairing. It has all been a well meaning fantasy, Jungle Man began to think, feeling foolish that he had let himself be seduced by the dream of one day returning. And then John Connigan had entered the picture.

He had been discovered on a psychiatric ward by Doctor X, who had instantly recognized his value. Although it was apparent that Connigan had serious problems, and had a long history of mental illness, he was a friendly, gentle man, and it was equally obvious that he possessed deep secrets and enormous potential.

Connigan had three months earlier shot himself in the head after losing his job at a government research center. Never popular with his co-workers, who resented his brilliance and despised his obvious mental fragility, he had been the butt of incessant jokes and pranks. Every day turned into an endurance test for this quiet, troubled man, who was helpless before his tormentors.

One late Friday afternoon, he had been sent into the cadaver lab to retrieve some supplies, and they locked him inside. The lights were deliberately shut off in this windowless room, and for an entire weekend Connigan had to live among the cadavers, a dim red emergency light his only illumination. When they opened the door on Monday morning he was found sitting on a large counter, calmly eating a leg.

That ended his employment and led to his suicide attempt, a long rehabilitation, and eventually to Doctor X. Now he was allied with them, leading them in their formerly hopeless quest, a helpless giant given to mood swings and trancelike states. Jungle Man did his best to protect him, as did all of his followers.

Despite Connigan's internal hell, he remained scientifically dazzling. Doctor X and Mr. Natural, each of whom had advanced training in the sciences, seemed in awe of his genius. Within weeks he was producing one breakthrough after another. The mood at their little headquarters had gone from one of dejection to that of elation, as Connigan transformed the Final Crusade from a hopeless dream into a genuine plan of action.

Now they were on the verge of launching their attack, and it was all thanks to this sleeping man. Jungle Man closed his eyes, praying for success.

"What are you thinking about?" Mr. Natural asked him.

"Nothing. I think I'll get some sleep now. The next few days will be very difficult."

"Suit yourself," Mr. Natural said, shrugging. He blew into his cup and took a loud sip.

Jungle Man arose and slowly walked out of the room.

chapter 43

Dean lay on the mattress, staring at the ceiling. Shadows from the candles danced with each other above him. Frenchie sat on the floor, her back against the wall, biting a fingernail. The room was very quiet.

The two had lived for hours in this underground chamber, gently coexisting, but not really talking. Both appeared a little embarrassed at their earlier outburst of emotion, and in any event, nothing seemed to lend itself to conversation. Dean stole innumerable glances at her, noting again and again how attractive she was, looking again and again at her curves, which the candlelight seemed to accentuate. It's hopeless, he thought, she's too gorgeous for me, I wouldn't get to first base. I've never been good at this, I'm just not the sexy type. Anyway, she'd think I was crazy for even trying to flirt with her, here in this dungeon or whatever this place is.

The more he thought about her the more he tried to lose his desire, so that being alone with her wouldn't be so painful. When Frenchie stretched lazily, her honey colored skin glistening amidst the shadows, Dean closed his eyes. She's not that pretty, she's not that pretty, he kept saying to himself.

"Dean?"

"What?" he said with a start, surprised to hear her voice, anxious that she had somehow read his thoughts.

"What do we do now?"

Dean looked around and shrugged. "I guess we try to escape. Not that I know where we actually are."

"We've got to be underground," she said. "There's no heat or air conditioning and it's a little cool. Like a cave."

"I'll buy that. So we dig our way out of here."

"I'm ready when you are, boss."

"Why not. And I hereby designate you assistant boss," he said lightly.

She laughed. "You know, you're a nice person. You are."

He accepted her remarks with a smile, but inwardly he felt a pang of disappointment and sadness. From his experience, words like these were the romantic kiss of death; as far as he could tell, it was not possible to be nice and attractive at the same time. Finkel had once told him, women may marry men they like, but they sure as hell don't fuck them. Dean was inclined to agree.

"Thanks," he replied, trying to conceal his dejection.

"No, really, you're all right. You don't act like a doctor."

"I'm a person. Being a doctor is just a job."

"You wouldn't know it from talking to other doctors. They all treat you like you're fourteen years old."

"That's their problem, not mine," he said wearily. "Believe it or not, it's their loss more than anyone else's."

"You okay? Did I say something wrong?"

"No, no, everything's fine. So, how about we explore this place. It shouldn't take very long."

They both stood up. Dean looked away from Frenchie. She wants it like that, she'll have it like that, he thought, realizing how petty he was sounding, and how ridiculous his emotions were in view of what was going on all around them.

Together they walked the perimeter of the makeshift cell, at times side by side. As he walked he willed things back into perspective. I have a life on the outside, he said to himself. Believe it or not, this is not my only world, as difficult as that may feel right now.

"I don't see any way out," he said after they had completed their second round of inspection. "There's no trap door, no windows, just a small drain on the floor here. As of now, I'm stumped."

"So what do we do?" Frenchie asked, looking at him earnestly.

"Honestly, I think we're doing it. Listen, do you want to talk? At least it will take our minds off this craziness."

"What do you want to talk about," she said absently, grimacing at the layers of dust in the corner.

"Well, tell me something about yourself. How do you know Toot and Godfrey. What do you do for a living. Stuff like that."

She sat down on the edge of the mattress, looking away.

"I used to be rough and tough, and I used to be bad," she said distantly. "Now I'm just boring."

"What do you mean?" Dean asked, sitting down on the other side of the mattress.

"You really want to hear?"

"Yeah, definitely."

"I guess you might as well," Frenchie said. "I hate lies, and making believe you're something you're not is a lie."

She turned to fully face him, sitting with her legs crossed.

"I'm thirty-eight, and have a twenty year old son who I haven't seen since birth. I used to do dope and once I even walked the streets so I could buy the dope. That was a long, long time ago. I don't think I've even been on a date in the last five years, and I haven't even had a drink in ten. I've known Godfrey since I was three—we lived in the same apartment house. We're like family. He's been more like a real brother than … I live with my mother and drive a school bus. It's a very simple life, but at least I don't think I'm going to hell anymore. Do you want to know anything else?"

"Wow. I'm sorry, you didn't have to … how come you quit doing what you were doing? If I may ask."

"You can ask. After a while I started feeling worse and worse about it. Towards the end I had trouble looking in the mirror. I always knew it was wrong, but for a while it was fun, and when you're young, fun's what it's all about. After a while, though, the shame caught up to me, and I just stopped.

"These days I just work and go straight home. That's it, that's my life. I just wish I had gone to school because now, well, there's nothing to do. I read lots and lots of books. I read every day, sometimes for hours."

"You must have some great stories of your own," Dean said uneasily.

"A few, but they aren't so great. They're just wild, mostly about the extremes people can go to. And they're fading with time, which is good. When I do think about them, which is hardly ever, it's hard to believe that was me. It was a whole other life."

She straightened her legs out before her and bent over, easily touching her toes.

"Boy, your muscles get stiff doing nothing," she said. "Anyway, I went along with Godfrey partly to look up my brother, who I haven't seen in two years, and partly for a change of pace. Everything's become so routine, it's like I needed to stretch a little. I guess I got more than I bargained for."

"Things sure aren't routine now," Dean said.

"I'll say. Here I am, locked in a dungeon with a good looking doctor. Indians with knives are running around, people dying all over the place ..."

"Good looking, huh?" Dean murmured, half to her and half to himself.

"So what about you, cell-mate," she said. "You know me cold now. What's your tale of woe?"

"It won't match yours. I'm forty six, no kids, divorced, hurting a little from the alimony, and I guess a little depressed. I hate to say it, but I came along partly for the excitement too.

"I spent the best years of my life trying to become a doctor, studying to become a doctor, or being one. I don't think too much in the ER anymore, a lot of it's just instinct and reflex now. I'm in the all-work, no-play phase of my life now. It's lonely. Most of it is my fault. I'm lousy with people and even worse with relationships. I have a list of things to do that would boggle your mind, all different types of adventures. But so far I haven't even started on the first item, and I think I'm too old to try out most of them anyway. Overall, I think I'm a little on the boring side. That's me in fifty words."

"You a bore?" she asked. "No way. You're glamorous compared to me."

She turned to him, her eyes almost shining in the darkness. As hard as he tried, he couldn't resist looking into them. He willed himself to move an inch in her direction. To him it seemed dazzling and bold. She didn't move. Dean's heart began to pound, as fear came over him. He was furious at himself. I'm middle aged and still afraid of girls, he thought. Dean, you are helpless and hopeless in equal parts..

"You okay?" she asked, not taking her eyes off him.

"Yeah, it's just that … ah, never mind."

"What? What is it?"

"It was just a question. It's not important."

Frenchie rolled to her side, propping herself up with an elbow. "It is important. Ask me."

With all his might, marshaling every ounce of his flagging courage, Dean looked at her.

"Would you let me kiss you?"

Her lips parted ever so slightly, and with the barest of motions she nodded yes.

He reached over and gently pulled her onto the mattress, marveling at her softness. They kissed. It was the most natural sensation he had ever felt and jolts of sheer happiness surged through his body. For a moment he felt as if he would faint, but he didn't, and he pulled her against him. They lay down on the mattress, their arms tightly wrapped around each other, no longer two lost people but now a passionate couple acting as one.

Minutes later, when he entered her, he had the feeling of finally, at long last, being home. I belong here, with her, he thought. God, as you are my witness, she makes me alive.

They made love again and again, each time better than the time before, each moment of passion greater than the one preceding it, each time leaving them feeling closer to the other. When finally they finished, they lay in each other's arms, exhausted and ecstatic, and when they drifted off to sleep, they dreamed of each other. The underground shadows danced with delight to the silent music of the flickering candle.

chapter 44

It seemed as if they had been in the underground chamber forever, although Dean reckoned the time to have been just a few days. Without clocks, windows or the remotest sight or sound from the outside, they lived by their own rhythms, and to their amazement, they were totally happy.

Sitting opposite her on the mattress, Dean told her everything that had happened over the past few weeks, from meeting Connigan to the recent deaths in the ER. Frenchie listened intently, seeming to absorb everything he said. She was particularly interested in his descriptions of all the people he worked with and what their reactions were to everything that had happened.

"Mr. Natural, he's one of them. So is someone else in your group, I'd bet on it."

Dean kept quiet, thinking of all his friends. Helen, the gentle woman with the faraway eyes? Finkel, the ultimate cynic? Ehler? He was known in the ER as 'the machine', so great was his logic and scientific reasoning.

The mere thought that any of his friends could actually be a deadly foe deeply upset him. He felt betrayed and horribly exposed. He turned to Frenchie. She was looking at him curiously. He smiled thinly at her.

"Here, look at this," he said, changing the subject. He pulled the copy of Connigan's book from his pocket. It was smeared with dirt, and the pages were starting to fray.

"What is it?" she asked, bewildered.

"Very strange stuff is what it is. It's all I have to go on, but I bet somewhere in these notes is the way to stop these fanatics."

Frenchie read the pages intently, seeming to concentrate on each word. Dean watched her, admiring her beauty. I can't believe she is all mine, he thought. After a few minutes, she suddenly put the book down and looked deeply into his eyes. Wordlessly, she moved towards him.

"How about a little study break?" she whispered.

"You know what they say about all work and no play," he whispered back, touching her face with his hand. With his other he tapped out the candle's flame. Total darkness engulfed them as their arms intertwined, and they became one yet another time.

After a while it seemed as if they could finish each other's sentences, and Dean got the impression of two lost puzzle pieces that somehow had been reunited. He couldn't take his eyes or hands off her, and to his continuing delight and astonishment, she passionately accepted each and every one of his advances.

"You really like me?" he asked her. "As in, 'really' like me? I'm not too nice?"

"You're my shining knight," she told him. "You're everything I always wanted in a man, and I'm gonna stay with you. If you let me."

She pulled herself to him and then looked up, staring deeply into his eyes. Dean felt her hotness, and put his arms around her.

"You're so many good things wrapped into one," she whispered.

Dean, who had spent his lifetime at arm's distance, held on to her tightly. Who are you, he thought, you make me feel alive for the first time ever. You who make me feel energized and peaceful at the same time …

"I'm never going to leave you," he said. "Frenchie, I'm going to play this hand."

She smiled up at him.

"You took the words right out of my mouth."

chapter 45

"Mate!"

Frenchie looked up from their makeshift chessboard, triumphantly. Dean frowned. He had taught her the game three days earlier, and she was again easily beating him.

"That's thirteen games to two," she said with sweet coyness.

"Excuse me, but I won three games," Dean objected.

"I accidentally knocked the board over," she protested. "Surely you can't penalize me …"

"World Federation rules. I have no choice. And now that I'm warmed up, you are officially in serious trouble."

"You've had it," Frenchie said, shaking her head. "I'm gonna whip your butt so bad …"

"Can we stop grandstanding and get on with the next …"

She interrupted with a kiss. He closed his eyes, basking in the sensation. After a few seconds, she gently pulled away.

"You ought to see me at puzzles," she said proudly. "In the last year there wasn't one that was too hard, even in the Sunday papers. It just took a while to memorize all the capitals and rivers. Now I do 'em every day, it's a piece of cake."

"Puzzles?"

"Yeah, they're fun. I started doing them on the subway. I do at least two or three a day. Lately my thing has been sudoku and code games— all that stuff. My other big hobby is history. The ancient Greeks, the

Crusades—they're my favorite, by the way—Napoleon, the African empires. You name it, I've read about it. I'm also into literature. Last week I finished *Doctor Faustus* by Marlowe. "

"Don't say anything but you could be one of the smartest people I've ever met," Dean said.

"I know I don't look smart, but I think I am," she said, turning serious. "Every night, after a long, hot bath for my back, it's straight to reading. Like the saying goes, before I die I want to read just two more books—per day. Any subject, any story.

"It'd be so good to, you know, have one more chance. Just one more. I swear this time I'd stay in school, and I'd never stop. God, there's so much in the world to learn about."

"I guess it was tough where you grew up," Dean said carefully.

"Where I grew up they beat up the smart kids," she said, staring distantly at the gray walls. "They were treated almost like traitors."

"Where I went to school the smartest kids were the big shots," Dean said, surprised.

"All the 'cool' people dropped out," Frenchie continued. "It makes me sad to even think about it. Being cool back then really meant you cashed in your chips early, you know, just so you could strut for a while. The bad part of it was, that's what the outside expected of us, and worse, that's what we expected of ourselves—you'd look in the mirror and you wouldn't see many choices, and most of them were bad. It was, like, what costume will I wear today. The big guys tried out for sports. For the rest, well, there was crime, welfare or if you were lucky, a civil service job."

"Sounds really bleak," Dean said.

"That was the world. What a waste. There were some bright ones, too. You'd see them just sort of fall off to the side of the road, so to speak, as they got older. Godfrey, he was, is, the smartest guy I ever met. I swear he'd have cured cancer by now if he'd had the chance. Killer, too."

"Who?" Dean asked, squinting at her.

"Not important," she said quickly.

"Anyway, it is horrible," Dean said defensively. "I tell you, I don't know how things got so bad."

Frenchie quickly touched his hand.

"Oh, it's not you," she said. "It's the system. As for me, I just don't think about it much. That's the way things are, and they're getting better. Anyway, like I was saying, puzzles and codes are my thing. With my smarts and your toughness we're a cinch to get out of here."

"Toughness," Dean said with a laugh. "Listen, I hate to say this, but I'm not a tough guy."

"You're big and tall, and I saw what you did to those Indians, or whatever they were. You're tough all right."

"Well, if I am, I don't know it."

"You ever hunt or fish?"

"Never hunted. Killing for fun just isn't my cup of tea. As for fishing, yeah. I've done it, but a lot of it is just to get outside and look at the scenery without looking weird. I don't try to catch anything. When I do, if I haven't half-killed it getting the hook out, I throw it back."

They both chuckled.

"Yeah, I'm a real killer," Dean murmured to himself.

Frenchie suddenly turned serious. For a moment Dean thought he has said something to offend her and played back in his mind their conversation. Then Frenchie spoke.

"The leader of the Death Masters, his name is Killer. He's so evil you have no idea. He's even hunted people. Godfrey told me that his thing was to pick out someone he wanted to kill, someone he never met before and follow him, without his knowing it, and then catch him and beat him to death."

Dean shivered. "That's the sickest thing I've ever heard. And Godfrey was in that gang?"

"In it? He *started* it, almost twenty years ago. Killer was his number two man."

"That's just great. He's worse than this Killer person?"

"No, never. He didn't have the meanness," Frenchie said. "For him, it was more like a business and a way to get respect. He was famous around here. A lot of people still look up to him. But things change. He's a good man now."

"Yeah, what does he do?" Dean asked warily.

"He's a maintenance man at the private school I work for."

Dean nodded, and smiled tightly. It was painful to think of Godfrey, who he secretly admired, who certainly once possessed considerable power and prestige, spending his life mopping floors and unclogging toilets.

"Frenchie, listen. Assuming this craziness is just someone's hallucination, or if it's stopped, or something, when we get out of here, I'll get you into school. I swear, whatever you want to study, I'll help and support you."

She touched his hand gently.

"That would be very nice. I'd like that."

"I would do it. You're the best thing that's ever happened to me."

"Even though I'm who I am? And did what I did?"

Dean paused. He was trying to find something sweet to say, but deep within him a voice said, no more games, go for broke.

"What," Frenchie asked, biting her lip. "Now you've got me all worried."

Dean looked at her, his mind racing. He was starting to get dizzy. I swear we were made for each other. Don't be a fool and play by other people's rules. Make your own for a change, and be happy.

"I'm in love with you," he said.

He kissed her. Frenchie barely moved, until Dean put his arms around her. Then she hugged him as hard as she could. They held each other in the semi-blackness of the still room, totally consumed with each others' presence.

"Am I your man, Frenchie?" Dean asked, kissing her neck.

"Yeah, and I'm your woman, Dean," she whispered, staring at the candle's flame. "Do with me what you want."

Their shadows again merged into one, gently, briefly, swaying on the wall. Frenchie reached down and tapped out the flame with a finger. The darkness was full and sweet.

chapter 46

Hours later they lay on the mattress. Dean held Frenchie, who was curled against him, sleeping. Occasionally she'd murmur something in her sleep, and he'd watch her face, marveling at its soft lines.

It's amazing how this has actually been a good thing for me, he thought, kissing Frenchie on the forehead. She mumbled and snuggled closer. But it's time to leave this place. I wonder what's going on above ground. This Doctor X is way off base. To find paradise you don't have to destroy everything and start from scratch—you just need someone you love.

As he drifted off to sleep, he thought to himself, over and over, when we get out of here, we are going to be very happy.

The next thing he knew he was being nudged in the ribs. Bolting upright, he looked around, for a while not remembering where he was.

Frenchie was sitting next to him. She was wearing his shirt, holding Connigan's book next to the candle.

"Dean, parts of this are in code. Some stuff is just plain crazy, as far as I can tell, but a lot's in code. It's not that hard, either, you just have to be able to break into it."

Dean stared at her quizzically.

"This I've got to hear."

"Okay, listen to this.

> *Fearsome Unknowns Come Knocking,*
> *Implicitly Threatening.*
> *Everyone Needs Dying. I Tremble*
> *Amid Nature's Divination,*
> *Awaiting Lush, Luxuriant*
> *Growth, In Verdant Ecstasy, Under Peonies."*

"Well, it's a poem," Dean said, perplexed. "It sounds sort of nice, I guess, in a gloomy way. What's so unusual? It doesn't mention any of this stuff."

"In code it does," Frenchie said. "The man who wrote it capitalized the first letter of each word. If you put them all together it reads like this:

> *Fuck it, end it, and ',all give up.*

Dean's eyes widened. "You're kidding."
"Look for yourself."
Dean scanned the words, and then looked at Frenchie with awe.
"You're not kidding! You're a genius," he said.
"I wish. No, it's just a simple thing. It gets more complicated."
"What else do you see?" Dean asked.
"Little things. Here's one: ',

> *I Lay On Velvet Eternity,*
> *Yearning Over Utopia,"*
> *Passing O'er Nirvana's Yellow"*

"'I love you, pony,'" Dean translated for himself. "That doesn't make sense. Except that he mentions ponies several times in the book."

"Here's another one that doesn't make sense," Frenchie said.

> *Looking At Catastrophe,*
> *Often Pensive, Ever Restive, Overly Nervous"*

"'Lac Operon,'" Dean said, the hair rising on his scalp. He had started growing happily complacent with Frenchie; now, the icy reality of what was going on crashed back to his consciousness.

"What did you say?" Frenchie said.

"Nothing. Everything. It's a process that activates, or deactivates, our genetic code. At least in bacteria. Connigan implied he found the human equivalent in the book."

"This disease strikes our genes?"

"That's what it looks like."

"This is not your typical RNA or DNA virus, is it?"

"You know about viruses?"

"I've read about them."

There was a crumbling sound. Though it was barely audible, it was the first external noise they had heard since being locked up, and it sounded like an avalanche. They froze, wondering if the walls were starting to collapse.

"What was that?" Dean whispered.

Frenchie looked around, attempting to trace the source.

"It came from that floor drain over there," she whispered back, pointing to the center of the room.

"I'll take a look."

"Dean, be careful."

"What's the worst that could happen, I'm just going from here to there," he said half jokingly. "I think I should make it."

Stuffing the papers in his pocket, he got off the mattress. Wordlessly, they both dressed. Then Dean walked over. He tapped the drain with his foot. There was another crumbling sound.

"It seems sort of solid," he said, half to himself.

"I don't want there to be a cave-in or anything," Frenchie said. "This building is ancient."

"It seems okay enough," Dean said, tapping the drain with a foot. "I bet this thing leads somewhere."

He started jumping on the section of the floor by the drain, each blow from his feet producing more and more noise from below. The ground around him seemed to loosen, the century-old floor cracking all around them.

"Dean, be careful!" Frenchie said anxiously.

"Don't worry. Now let's formulate a plan …"

He crashed through the floor, as the entire section gave way, plummeting nearly six feet, landing on what seemed to be a giant pile of ash and dirt. There was an explosion of powder in the dimly lit space from the impact. He rolled off the pile, coughing violently. Above, he could hear Frenchie screaming.

"I'm not hurt, I'm not hurt," he said between coughs.

She ran to the opening, peering down, holding a candle.

"Are you okay?" she gasped.

"Yeah, just some scratches. Thank God for these ashes, they saved my neck. It's probably stuff they swept through that grate for who knows how many years. This must be some sort of storage room or passageway. Hey, Frenchie, there's a light about twenty yards down."

"Wait for me," she said.

She passed the candle down to Dean and started lowering herself down, letting herself swing from the edges of the gaping hole. Dean caught her when she let go, and she put her arms around him.

"I told you I'd find a way out," he said with a half smile.

She looked at him, concern in her eyes.

"Well, ready to escape?" he asked, lighting an extra candle and giving it to her. The flames washed waves of soft yellow over her face. Dean noticed she wasn't smiling.

"What's the matter, I told you we'd somehow get out …"

"You meant what you said up there right, right?" she asked quietly. "Was it all just a dream, or some desert island fantasy?"

Dean looked at her and nodded solemnly. "Yes, I meant every word," he said.

"It won't be easy," she said.

"Yeah, but I bet it's gonna be fun."

"Then I'm ready to escape. Take me out of here."

They looked around and both saw the old furnace at the same time, now little more than a rusted hulk of metal. Beyond it lay a long underground tunnel, one that seemed to travel on an upward incline towards the surface. Dean realized that they were in the building's furnace room, and that coal and ash used to be transported through the dark tunnel before them. At the tunnel's end there were outlined a few cracks of light.

Hunching themselves over, so as to fit in the small space, they started walking. Their candles flickered almost sadly, as if to know that they would soon go back to their usual obsolescence.

At the tunnel's end there was a thin layer of wood in front of them. It was all that separated them from the outside world. What sounded like a truck rumbled by. To Dean it sounded like rolling thunder.

Dean and Frenchie squeezed each other's hands. They were excited that their imprisonment was over, but sad that the private world they shared, with its total dedication to each other, was going to end forever. Whatever was to happen after this, things would never be the same.

"Remember, I meant every word I said," Dean told her, squeezing her hand.

She nodded at him, a frightened look on her face.

With all his might, he crashed into the wall, which shattered before him. With a shout they burst through the opening and into the deserted street, startling several stray dogs, who ran away yelping.

They charged down the street, half blinded by the midday brightness. The urban squalor all around seemed to be practically ultra modern after their dungeon-like experience. A few people looked up at them, and then away, seeing little more than two dirty street people scurrying nowhere in particular.

Several blocks later, Frenchie signaled for them to stop. They staggered a few more feet, then sat down on the hood of an abandoned car, gasping for breath. They were in a crowded neighborhood now, with children on their way to school, shoppers and honking cars. Each sighed with relief. They had escaped.

chapter 47

They quickly left the neighborhood. Frenchie knew the area intimately and led them through all sorts of short cuts. Dean no longer attracted the same sort of look that he had days before—his clothes were now ripped, he badly needed a shave, and he was caked with soot. Indeed, it was only when they shortly entered the adjacent, more affluent area that he was startled by the suspicious, hostile glares he received. He turned to Frenchie in bewilderment. She looked amused.

"Now you know," she said. "So where to, my little hoodlum?"

"Back to my place to clean up. I wonder what day it is."

They had been holding hands on the crowded thoroughfare. Impulsively, Dean grabbed Frenchie and kissed her. They swayed on the sidewalk, holding onto each other. Dean sensed the shock they were creating among the people hurriedly walking around them. He knew it was more than his being disheveled. Once he would have been paralyzed with self-consciousness, but no longer. That's for them to work out, not me, he thought.

When they resumed walking, it was at a more leisurely pace. He searched in vain for a sign of impending trouble. Everything appeared the same. No one seemed sick, the buses blared, people rushed. If it wasn't for the mark on his neck, and this woman by his side, he would have sworn that he had just dreamt the whole thing.

He decided to call Ehler and walked over to a corner pay phone—he was grateful, there weren't many left these days. Frenchie dutifully waited, drifting over to a nearby store window and looked at the display. Ehler wasn't home. He called Finkel. Again, no answer. Dean hesitated, and then decided to call the ER. He had hoped to avoid this because somewhere in there, lurking in the shadows, was Doctor X.

The phone rang endlessly, as usual. While he waited for someone to pick up he snuck glances at passersby's newspapers, trying to find out the date and any recent events. Finally, someone answered.

"Emergency," Gloria drawled. It was common practice in the ER for any available person to pick up a ringing phone.

"Gloria, it's Doctor Miller," he nearly shouted.

"Doctor Miller, where you been?" she said, her voice suddenly sounding sharp, and to Dean's ears, a little suspicious. "Everyone's looking for you."

"Who's looking for me?" he said, annoyed at her tone. "Listen, are either Doctor Ehler or Doctor Finkel there?"

"No one's here. Just some new docs. If anyone comes in, where you gonna be?"

"I'll be at home. Just tell them I called. If you see Carol or Julie, tell them also."

"Yeah, no problem," she said distantly.

Dean hung up, frowning. He had never liked Gloria, especially since their recent confrontation, and this brief conversation he found unsettling.

"Let's go to my place, it's right around the corner," he said to Frenchie, trying to put the housekeeper out of his mind. They resumed walking.

"What are we going to do?" she asked. "What's the plan?"

"We make a few more attempts at alerting the authorities. If that doesn't work, we do it ourselves."

"Do what ourselves?"

"Find out where their secret place is and prevent them from doing this."

"Doing what. Where is this place?"

"I have no answer to either of your questions. You're the codebreaker. Maybe you'll tell me."

"And if you did find this place, is it possible that those jungle people are guarding it?"

"I would imagine so," Dean replied.

"So you don't know who or where your enemy is, what he's going to exactly do, and on top of that, he's heavily guarded. And we are going to stop him. Does that pretty much sum it up?"

"Well, if you want to put it like that. But remember, we have the book. Plus the element of surprise."

"I'm with you all the way. Those bad guys don't have a chance." She put her hands to her brow and shook her head, smiling in spite of herself.

They entered the lobby of his apartment. The doorman's mouth dropped when he saw Dean in his ragged condition.

"What day is today, George?" Dean asked.

"Thursday," the man stammered.

"God, six days. Amazing how time flies, isn't it. By the way, George, may I borrow your paper?"

The doorman nodded dumbly, speechless, and handed over his newspaper. They walked into the lobby and waited by the elevator, ignoring George's stares.

Dean kissed Frenchie again. "He's cool, I take great care of him every Christmas. And now, let's go upstairs for some strategy."

She snapped to attention and saluted him.

"Lead the way, general."

They immediately ripped off their clothes when they entered his apartment, throwing them in a pile by the window. Then they ran into the bathroom and took a long, hot shower together. Minutes later they fell gratefully into bed, where they made intense, passionate love. Then they took another steaming shower.

Afterwards, Frenchie watched Dean shave, then shooed him out, assigning him to make some coffee.

"I feel like making myself up a little, okay?"

"Fine with me," he said. "Maybe I'll call the ER again, too."

Outside, he dried off and dressed, astounded at how clean he felt. He walked over to his little kitchen and went ahead with the coffee, making it strong. But I'll show her some mercy, Dean thought with a smile, I'll just shoot for samurai. After adding a little milk that was still, just barely, fresh, he sat down at his table and opened the newspaper, scanning it for some hint of what was going on.

He had gotten to the movie section and had not seen as much as one story on any type of illness. How can that be, he wondered. There's not even any mention of the deaths in the ER.

He walked over and sat on the bed, and plugged his long dead cell phone into its charger. He punched in the ER's number. This time his call was quickly answered.

"ER, Miss Shea speaking."

"Julie, it's Dean. How is …"

"Dean! Where the hell are you?"

He was stunned at her outburst. He had never known Julie to raise her voice.

"Why're you so upset? Didn't Gloria give you my message that I'm home?"

"No, as a matter of fact she just walked out, and told us all to drop dead. Forget her. Dean, where have you been! I've been sick with worry. Are you okay?"

"They're not letting me work in the ER so I went out of town, in a way. It was sort of a last minute decision. What's up?"

"The world's gone crazy, that's what's up. First, you vanish, without so much as a goodbye. No one knew where you went. Then Finkel and Carol disappear. Someone called and left a message for them, saying they ran off to get married. Good for them, I swear they were made for each other, but not like that. The way they did it, it was not like them. Then Ehler walks out of the ER, I mean, just *walks* out and doesn't come back. He supposedly leaves a message in the ER office, saying he quits. Quits. Ehler, the most stable human in the world. I called his house ten times, but no answer.

"Tannenbaum's gone, too. He came looking for you last week, got into this horrible fight with Helen and left right after that. His secretary said he left for another conference. Dean, things are so weird. Thank God you're okay."

"Is Helen around?" Dean asked, very concerned.

"She's on vacation. At least that was scheduled."

"Julie did you speak to anyone about this, like the police?"

"I spoke to those creeps. They didn't really see anything wrong. You're on vacation. A man and a woman get married. Someone quits, someone goes on a conference. No crimes are committed, no complaints are filed. Oh, and speaking of crime, I was mugged three days ago."

"No."

"Oh, yeah. It was the scariest thing. I finished my shift and was walking to the bus stop when four guys jumped me. I mean, literally jumped me. They knocked me to the ground, but I tell you, I fought like mad. I didn't know I had it in me. They all ran off, without a dime. All I got was a few scratches on my neck. It's almost like a burn, it's the strangest thing ..."

"Julie, were they Indians?"

"What? Dean I didn't really look ... maybe. I don't know—it all happened so fast. Why did you ask that?"

Dean half smiled. It sounded like she's been protected. If I had to save someone, it would be her, he thought. Doctor X not only knows her, like I suspected, but he has good taste.

"Julie, listen good. This will sound bizarre but you have to believe me. This whole thing sounds like the Doctor X conspiracy. Finkel, Carol, Ehler, they knew too much, they may have been silenced. For some reason you were spared, that's what those marks on your neck are. The plotters seem to be centered in our hospital. They could be anyone. They caught me but I escaped. I'm going to get them, I swear."

There was a silence at the other end of the phone, and then he thought he heard the sound of Julie laughing. Suddenly he realized she was crying.

"Oh Dean, I'm so sorry, I really am. I always thought you were the greatest. God, if I could only help you."

He was momentarily confused by her tone, then realized that she was treating him as if he had gone mad.

"Julie, please, this is on the level," he said.

"Dean, can you stop by the ER?"

"I don't think so. Now listen to me, this is what I want you to do ..."

Suddenly there were outside voices—it was clear that Julie was talking to someone else. The receiver was muffled by her hand as she spoke heatedly. There was a clanging sound as the phone apparently fell from her hands. Another person seemed to grab it.

"Doctor Miller, ~~I presume~~ how the hell are you?"

It was Mr. Natural.

Dean said nothing. He began to tingle with fear.

"Doctor Miller, I know you're there."

"Yes, hello, how are you," Dean answered, trying to sound formal and calm at the same time.

"You don't sound too good, Doc, I think you need a checkup. I'll be more than glad to come pick you up. What's your address?"

"Thanks, but I'd rather not …"

"Don't thank me, it's my pleasure. I'll be right …"

"I'm at Finkel's apartment, I let myself in," Dean said quickly. "Tell Julie I'll be over in about two hours. Wait for me in the ER, you and I should have a little talk."

Mr. Natural started to protest, but Dean gently nested the phone into its cradle. At that moment Frenchie walked out, rubbing herself with a towel.

"Who was that on the phone," she asked.

"I think one of the bad guys. We don't have too much time."

She walked over to him, dropping the towel. She had used some of his ex-wife's makeup that had been left behind, which Dean found particularly arousing. He couldn't get over how beautiful she was.

"Let me get this straight," he said, holding her, his hands resting on her hips. "You're really all mine?"

"Yup."

"You know, I always figured that everything averages out, you know, the good times and the bad times. So I figured the pendulum would eventually swing my way again. But I never thought it would swing this good."

"Yeah, pendulums are funny that way."

She put her arms on his shoulders and gently pushed him down on the bed.

chapter 48

Frenchie studied Connigan's book while Dean lay in bed. He was nervously studying the ceiling, not knowing what to do. They'd been in his apartment for nearly an hour, and he sensed it was time to escape— but where to, and from whom? Suddenly, she sat up, as if making mental calculations.

"What's going on," he asked.

"It's interesting. Jungle Man's in here, even the part about human experiments. They seem to work out of a small, purple house on Jupiter Street. That shouldn't be too hard to find. And it's not all that hard, this code, some parts are downright easy. You just have to know how to break into his style. I don't like calling people names, but he does sound crazy. The biggest thing, though, is that he keeps referring to a park."

Dean looked at her.

"Go on."

"Little Bear Park. Where is it?"

"Upstate, a bit of a drive," he said, perplexed.

"Maybe that's their headquarters, right?"

"That's a bit of a stretch. It's pretty remote, actually. There's nothing like buildings or laboratories around. As far as I remember it has lots of trees and not much else, except for some small mountains and some caves, some long ones. I used to camp up there a lot. It's huge; I wouldn't even know where to start looking."

"So, then maybe we should all go to the Jupiter house and check that out."

243

"It beats just sitting here ... what do you mean 'all of us?'"

"Well, we'll need Toot, he knows these people. And Godfrey, for protection. He's a pro."

"A pro what? Come on, he ditched us in some abandoned building. We ought to shoot him for desertion, not give him another chance. He and Toot, the great 'defenders of doctors.' The only good thing about what they did is that they left us alone, so we could be together."

He paused, thinking about his words.

"I guess I do owe them a drink when I see them" Dean said, grinning in spite of himself.

Frenchie smiled, looking very cute in his shirt, which was loosely draped around her..

"Yeah, maybe it was meant to be," she said. "But there had to be other reasons, there had to be. You do know that we were outnumbered and would have been killed if we fought back. Besides, Godfrey's not allowed to carry a gun, he's a convicted felon."

"Why am I not surprised."

"And Toot's one of them. He's from one of those jungle tribes. I don't know if he's even allowed to fight against his own kind."

"Then why in God's name do we need them now?" Dean asked.

"If this place is the real thing, then we'll need all the help we can get. Godfrey would never let you get hurt. Not after he gives his word. I grew up with him. His sister is my best friend. Even in that building, I knew that he would have protected us if he thought we were in danger. Besides, your friends are gone, so we all have left are mine. Let me call him, please."

"All right, if you say so. Just tell them, no funny business this time."

She walked over to the table and picked up the phone. Dean picked up the tattered book and flipped through the pages. He turned to the section *The Words of Doctor X.*

Despite the turmoil of the past few days, it still gave him chills to see the words penned in blood. He shuddered at seeing them again. It's hard to believe that this piece of writing may change the world, he thought. The ancient civilizations, the Renaissance, religion, philosophy, science, everything will vanish, as if they never existed. They'll leave no memory, no legacy. All the hard work that created them will have been for naught. All that will remain will be trees, tigers and a few primitive tribes.

He stared hatefully at the words, cursing the author, images of his family and friends flickering in his mind. He looked at the first few sentences.

> *At a crossroads we are, did you know? Midnight is either the end of the day, or it's the beginning, and we straddle it. On the breaking back of Mother Nature we have ridden to the final chapter . Full of greed, empty of vision, except maybe to rape another planet. Moon malls, can you see it? Eve looks down at her lost paradise and cries acid tears.*

There's something funny about these words, he thought, there's something here. Everything looks too contrived. Maybe there's a code here as well.

He tried the first letters of each word, then the last. Nothing made sense. Then, as if struck with lightning, he saw it.

> *At midnight, on full moon eve.*

You have to look at the first word of each sentence, he realized. He grabbed a piece of paper and rapidly jotted down a message. He soon had a poem.

> *At midnight, on full moon eve,*
> *In the little bear park in May,*
> *By blue spot a spell we'll weave*
> *So the world can begin to play. "*

Dean read it again and again, and grabbed a desk calendar. There was a full moon tonight. Then he looked at Frenchie. She just hung up, a look of exasperation about her.

"They're doing it tonight," he said excitedly. "At Little Bear Park, upstate. And it's going to be at the blue diamond campsite—there are cabins you can rent. I know that place. Frenchie, we have about six hours."

She looked at him while he wrote down the information on a piece of paper.

"To do what?" she asked nervously.

"I'm not sure, but we have to go there. Forget the house on Jupiter—it's probably empty by now. We're going to meet these people in the woods. What about your friends?"

"Listen, Godfrey's not at work, he's off today, and he doesn't have a cell phone. I've got to go get him. We wouldn't have a chance without him. Dean, this is serious. Those bad guys are gonna eat us alive."

"Okay, if it makes you feel better," Dean said tightly, trying to mask his growing fear. "Let's go get Godfrey."

"No, I'll go alone, you'd get killed if you went where he lives," she said quietly. "Even Godfrey couldn't save you. I belong there, they don't even notice me."

Dean could sense the strain in her voice.

"Listen, meet us on the steps of the main post office, the big one in midtown, in about one hour," she said carefully. "I'm betting on them being home. Wait for us if you get there first. We'll go straight to this place from there."

The thought of her leaving upset him. It seemed natural by now to spend every moment with her.

"You'll be okay, Frenchie? Shouldn't I go with you?"

She beamed at him.

"I'll be fine from now on. I got a boyfriend."

They hugged each other as hard as they could, kissing each other's necks. Dean was nearly high from the affection he felt for her. The differences between them, which once he would have thought enormous, now seemed trivial and distant. We're not the same, he thought, it's better than that. We're two perfectly fitting pieces of the same puzzle.

"I'll miss you," he whispered, half to himself.

The afternoon sun was starting to soften, and the sky outside his window turned a creamy yellow, with hints of pink and orange. It bathed his apartment in pastel shades. Dean's heart started to pound. I don't want this world to end, he thought, I just found my place in it. Please, don't let this be the last night. Please, don't let all of this happen.

He held her tightly, afraid to let go, knowing that in some way the fight had just begun, and would end only when he finally crossed paths with his now sworn enemy.

Gently, she released herself from his grasp. There was determination in her eyes.

"I'll see you," she said. "And you're gonna do it."

"Do what," he asked apprehensively.

"You'll know it when you see it, darling, and I'll be with you. I'm always going to be with you. We'll figure it out."

chapter 49

Miles away from the city, Jungle Man faced his followers, who sat in a semicircle before him. They were in a large chamber deep inside a mountain, having walked several hundred yards through a narrow, twisting cave. Several torches illuminated the area, which was bare except for a huge ceramic vat that rested on a ledge by the far wall. Beneath the ledge, between the vat and the wall, lay a clear mountain pool, its water gently bubbling and swirling as it formed an underground stream, to begin a hundred mile journey towards the ocean.

"We will soon begin to reverse five hundred years of injustice," he said to them. "Their sunset will be our dawn. We shall be ready."

The warriors nodded solemnly, fingering their weapons.

"Begin the process then, and report to your stations," he continued. "Any intruders are to be reported at once. Take no actions unless you are told to. But remember, once you are ordered to do something, do it and without question. If that means being told to kill, kill without passion, and without delay. You may use your guns until the sun goes down, then we fight with our traditional weapons."

The warriors nodded.

"The final crusade has begun. Tomorrow we will wake up in a new world."

The old man looked around.

"We will not fail. Now go to your posts."

The warriors stood up as one and slowly filed out. The wizened leader sat very still, thinking of the sun and how very much he missed it. He had kept his vow to not walk in the daylight for so many years. My life has been dark for so very long, he whispered silently to his gods. I have never asked for myself one thing, but I do so now, as I sit here surrounded by stone. I pray for the strength to awaken one more day, so that I may finally, once more, greet the light.

The sounds of the water trickling suddenly seemed to intensify. Jungle Man looked at it and smiled. "Thank you," was all he said.

chapter 50

With Frenchie gone, the apartment seemed cold and empty. Dean fidgeted anxiously. It somehow doesn't feel like home anymore. I should have gone with her, he thought.

He sat at his dining room table, half heartedly sipping some coffee. This hour is going to go on forever, he thought. What does one do with free time on the world's last day, anyway? I wish I could bring it up at the next code. It would put that last conversation to shame …

The phone rang.

He jumped. It was a second before he could control his thoughts. Then, embarrassed at his reaction, he gathered himself and picked up the receiver.

"Hello?"

"I had a hunch you'd be home, Doc," the voice said coldly.

It was Mr. Natural.

"What the hell do you want?" Dean hissed angrily;

"Is that any way to talk to old friends?"

"Damn you and damn your Doctor X!" he shouted into the phone, his voice quivering with emotion.

There was silence at the other end.

"You can't stop us," the guard finally said.

"We'll see about that. Fuck you a thousand times …"

There was a sound of the phone being gently hung up, and Dean found himself staring into a dead receiver. His hands began to shake.

He tried to calm himself by looking out the window. The sky was turning a rich shade of amber. They want a fight, he finally said to himself, they're gonna get a fight. Winner take all. First prize, third planet from the sun.

Dean went to his closet, put on a jacket, and removed a cloth laundry bag from a shelf. He quickly walked around his apartment, filling it. Kitchen knives, candy bars, anything he could think of. Out in five minutes, he said to himself, out in five, stuffing the bag with anything he imagined might come in handy.

While packing, he heard something scratching outside the door. In the past, he might not have noticed, or paid it any mind. But following his recent underground stay, with its thick, fragile stillness, the sound now seemed harsh and grating. Someone's in the hallway, he thought.

Quietly, he put down the half filled bag down and quickly put on his sneakers. Then he stood up, shoving his wallet and some money into a pants pocket. He softly went to the door to look through the peephole

As he approached, it crashed open, the door slamming into him. Dean reeled from the impact. Three men burst in. He stopped his backward motion, his mouth open with surprise. They ran up to him and hurled him violently into the opposite wall. He hit it with a cracking thud and fell to the ground.

Before he could process what was going on, he was dragged to his feet like a cloth doll. The men surrounded him in the middle of the room, one of them grabbing him from behind. Dean looked at them numbly, speechless with shock. The biggest man slapped him across the face several times, and then punched him in the stomach. The arms holding Dean let go, and he sank to his knees, blood dripping from both nostrils down his jacket and onto the floor.

Another pair of hands jerked him up again. Dean's eyes were wildly tearing and he could barely see anything. He had no idea what was happening, feeling only pure terror, reacting only as would an animal under attack from savage predators. His limbs were drained of all power, and he stood before them helplessly, completely defenseless.

His arms were pulled hard behind his back, his shoulders making crunching noises as they were twisted. He screamed in pain but in a distant way was grateful—it had the effect of washing away his confusion and focusing the situation. He realized now that several intruders had entered his apartment and that he was their captive.

The big man punched him several times in the face and then kneed him in the groin. Dean collapsed in agony, violently retching. He gagged and writhed frantically as two Death Masters stood over him.

The third man, known as The Snake, silently walked up and kicked him twice in the ribs. The other two men glowered down at him.

"Where is it?" the biggest man growled.

"Please, I didn't do anything," Dean panted, cowering on the ground.

"We didn't ask you what you 'did,'" the other man snarled, kicking Dean in the chest, rolling him onto his back. "We asked, where is it?"

Dean lifted his head. He was dizzy and was having trouble focusing his eyes. *I have to get out of here,* was all he could think about.

"Where's what? Please, I don't ..."

"Where's the book!" the biggest man shouted. He somehow appeared to be the leader. "Don't make me kill you."

"Please ..."

"Ghost, this is bullshit," the leader said. "Do your thing."

The man named Ghost bent over and started slapping Dean's face, then savagely twisted his ear. Dean howled in agony. He was bleeding from his mouth and nose, and now his ear felt as if it had been ripped off. He rolled over in disbelief.

"Diablo asked where the book is," Ghost said coldly.

"What book?" Dean cried out. "Don't hurt me."

"The Doctor X book," Diablo snapped, leaning over and grabbing Dean's collar, effortlessly lifting him off the ground. "I'm sick of waiting on you. I've been coming here for days ..."

"The kitchen," Dean gasped, pointed a trembling finger. "On the table."

"You lie, you die," the big man warned, releasing his grip. Dean crashed back onto the floor.

They walked into the other room, ignoring him. Dean rolled onto his side, desperately trying to catch his breath, and will the pain away. He could hear them pick up the book and flip through the pages.

"What's the big deal," he heard Ghost say. "Diablo, listen to this.

Yonder, Orderly Unicorns
Wander in Languid Luxury,
Dreaming in Ecstasy"

"Killer wants this?" Snake asked, bewildered. "What is it, a poem?"

"Don't care," Diablo growled. "Grab him and let's go. Snake, what you looking at?"

"The doc wrote something else," the gang member said, holding up a small piece of paper. "'Little Bear Park, tonight, blue diamond campsite.' I've heard of that park. Hey man, talk to me."

Snake walked over to him. Dean cringed as he approached, curling up on the floor.

"Something going down tonight? Talk to me."

"I don't know," Dean said, looking away. "Please, take what you want and leave me alone."

The Death Master grabbed him by the hair and pulled his face upwards, to within inches of his own. Dean writhed in pain.

"Don't do this," he whispered coldly. "I asked, is something going on? Does it have something to do with our men dying?"

Dean nodded fearfully. Somewhere deep inside of him a voice said, you can beat these guys you know, just not on their terms. With all his might he found his voice.

"The people who've been hunting you guys, the Doctor X people, they're meeting there tonight. For a celebration—a party—then they're gone forever. I'm not one of them, they're after me too …"

"What are they, another gang?"

"Sort of."

Snake let go of Dean's hair and walked back to the kitchen. Dean could see their shadows huddling through the open door as they whispered to each other. He lay on the floor, desperately trying to catch his breath.

"So Gloria was right all along," Diablo finally said out loud. "This Doctor X gang, we'll have to have a little talk with them. Ghost, get that guy and let's go. Killer wants to have some fun with him."

"Let me play with him first," Ghost protested. "Killer don't have to know."

"He's supposed to come back alive."

"Come on, I'm in the mood. This was too easy."

The big man was thoughtful for a moment.

"Just don't kill him," he warned. "And make sure he'll be able to talk. I'll fix something to eat, I'm hungry."

Diablo and Snake turned their attention to Dean's refrigerator, studying its contents. Dean thought he saw the one named Ghost walk over to the television and turn it on. An old movie blared. The assailant appeared to slip on leather gloves and walked towards him. They're going to kill me, Dean thought, either now or later. I don't have a chance, unless …

He looked around the room, planning his strategy. Distantly he noticed that his fear had gone—maybe they beat it out of me, he thought. I'm ready for you guys, I'm ready for your best shot. You just may kill me, but I'm going out with a fight. I took a bunch of martial arts a long time ago, hopefully something stuck.

He took some deep breaths and lay still.

"Hey mister, sit up and look at me," the Death Master said as he neared.

He approached, swaggering slightly. Through squinted eyes, Dean saw something metallic in the man's hand. He timed his move, holding his breath. Ghost bent down to grab him.

"I said sit …"

Dean shot up his hand up, the heel of his palm smashing the man on the point of his nose. Ghost grunted with pain, snorting blood. In an instant, Dean's hand slid over his face and with a lunging move he rammed his fingers deeply into both of the man's eye sockets. Instantly in shock, the Death Master fell forward. Dean caught him and eased him onto the floor. Carefully, he took a razor out of his twitching hand.

"Man, what you doing?" Snake called out in muffled tones, his mouth full of food. Dean heard him turn and walk out of the kitchen, headed for the living room. Quickly, he moved to the side of the kitchen door and waited.

Snake walked into the room, and froze at the sight of his friend lying on the floor, his face running with blood. At that moment Dean came up from behind, slashing his throat deeply . Snake's windpipe was instantly ripped open and he fell to the ground, hissing violently, furiously struggling for air, making gurgling, bubbling sounds as he choked on his own blood. Within seconds his motions became slower and slower. Dean watched him with horror.

"Hey? What's going on," Diablo bellowed from the kitchen. "What's with you guys. Keep it quiet, will you?"

Dean dropped the razor, quietly panting, desperately willing oxygen into his burning lungs. He wiped his blood smeared face with his sleeve. His nose continued to bleed, as did his cracked, swollen lips. Ignoring his injuries, he steadied himself for the fight with the big man. He grabbed the bag he had been packing, and pulled out a large knife.

"Guys?" Diablo asked again.

A gun battle between cowboys and Indians erupted on the television. The man he had slashed stopped moving. The blinded man was either unconscious, or dead. Dean froze with dread.

"Okay, what's the …"

The huge man slowly entered the room, his eyes fixing on his two fallen comrades. His lips mouthed words of disbelief, his eyes bulged in revulsion at their wounds. Then he turned to Dean and smiled icily. There was a look of sheer evil about him, mixed with a tinge of cold pleasure.

"Okay, motherfucker, let's rumble," he finally said.

I can't take this guy, he's going to kill me, Dean realized. He's bigger and stronger than me, I don't have surprise anymore, and he sure looks like he can fight. My knife won't even slow him down.

The blinded man twitched. Reflexively, Diablo turned to look at him. At that moment Dean made his move. He shot for the door, reaching it in an instant, threw it open and bolted out of sight. His surprised opponent watched him go, stunned for a few moments. Then with an almost visible shake of his head Diablo recovered, and ran into the hall, roaring out curses. The large man stopped halfway down the hall, looking around and listening in vain. Dean was gone.

Dean raced out of the building, bolting past a man leaning against an idling van, someone wearing clothing similar to what his assailants had worn. Gang colors, he realized. The man barely had time to look up as his intended prey rounded the corner.

Dean tore down the street, dropping the knife as he ran. His shirt was drenched with blood, most of it his. He ripped it off and tossed it in the gutter. Frightened pedestrians gaped at him as he went by. A couple of people who thought they knew him called out, but he didn't hear them. He was totally numb.

After staggering fifteen minutes more he found himself in a small, mostly empty park. He collapsed on a bench, gasping for breath. He had the outward appearance of a man gone crazy, and the few people who walked on by struggled to ignore him. After a while Dean stood up. His breathing was finally under control. He took a clean shirt out of his pack and slipped it on. The bag had blood all over it so he threw it away. Got to go, he said to himself, got to keep moving. There's no going back.

chapter 51

Frenchie, Toot and Godfrey didn't recognize Dean as he approached. They sat on the steps of the post office, passing around a large bag of fried potatoes, mulling over what Frenchie had told them.

"Me, I'm half rooting for Doctor X," Godfrey said. "You tell me what's so good about this world. The three of us, we're intelligent people, we're good people—and we're throwaways. Some of those doctors, they have half our brains, and they earn more in a day than we do in a month. Damn, I wish I had stayed in school."

"That's right," Toot said, licking his fingers.

"Listen, my future began at my conception, and ended the day I was born," Godfrey continued. "I lived in a different hotel almost every week, and there was a different man in the room just about every night. When they finally placed me with my aunt, her only rule was, 'you leave me alone, I leave you alone.' Hey, she was nineteen and had two kids of her own. I was running dope before I was ten. What do you think, Frenchie, your doctor boyfriend, when he was ten, what was he taking, tennis lessons or piano lessons?"

"He ain't bad, Godfrey."

"Don't get me wrong, I like him. He's actually pretty cool. French, this ain't a personal thing, and I don't mean to bore you with my life story ..."

"I know your life story, Godfrey, I was there, remember? My story ain't much better, or different," she said.

They exchanged smiles. They were like family to each other.

257

"It's all a geopolitical coincidence we're in this boat to begin with," Godfrey continued. "If the folks from our neck of the woods had the historical or cultural need to develop capitalism and military science, they would have. And then they would have taken over the world. And they probably would have messed things up just as bad. The only difference would have been that the shoe would just be on the other foot."

"At least we'd be the ones wearing it," Frenchie joked. They both laughed.

"The world today took centuries to get to this point, and it's going to take centuries more to fix," Godfrey said. "I can't say I'm very optimistic about the next few generations. You can't simply change society by passing a law."

He looked at his audience. Toot appeared not to have been listening. Frenchie was scanning the street. Undaunted, Godfrey decided to wrap up his discourse.

"Who knows, it just might be a good idea to wash everything clean and start over. Face it, things couldn't come out any worse for us."

"Toot, you agree with Doctor X?" Frenchie said. She was staring intently at a figure staggering down the street towards them.

"If Jungle Man wants it, then it must be a good thing. He once told me that the world is aging faster than we now, and will die before we do. Maybe this will stop things from getting to that point."

"No way," Frenchie said, distracted by the approaching man. She turned and pointed across the street. "Look at those children. Are you prepared to let them all die? Guys, this ain't a game. It's real-life versus real death. Personally, I'm on the side of life ... who the hell ... Oh, Lord!"

They all recognized Dean at once and rose to meet him. He nearly collapsed in their arms. They sat him down on the marble steps and surrounded him, as if they were corner men reviving their fighter between rounds.

"What happened," Frenchie blurted out, tears in her eyes. She was caressing his swollen face, which was red with dried blood. "I never should have left you."

"Three guys came into the apartment," Dean gasped. "They wanted the book. They were going to kidnap me."

"Man, they sure did a number on you," Toot said, impressed.

"I, I think I killed two of them," Dean stammered, his lower lip quivering. "I never hurt anyone before."

"Well, I must say, this is getting interesting," Godfrey said with a half smile.

"What hurts the most?" Frenchie asked.

"Everything."

"You're telling me that they didn't want money?" Godfrey asked, perplexed.

"They just wanted the book. The big guy, Diablo, he has it now. I had to give it up. They also know about the park."

"Of course, honey, don't worry about it," Frenchie said. She carefully put her arms around him and hugged gently, trying to hide her concern.

"Diablo," Godfrey repeated softly, a strange look in his eye.

"They had weird names. Snake, Ghost. They were the ones I killed. And they were going to bring me … they were going to bring me to someone named …"

Dean sat upright, fear in his eyes. He looked at Godfrey, and then at Frenchie. The two were exchanging stunned glances.

"They were going to take me to Killer. Did you have anything to do …"

"No," Godfrey simply said. "I'm on your side."

"Is Diablo as bad as his name?" Dean asked, wincing from the pain in his ribcage.

"Just about. He's a very violent man. The only one who can keep him in line is Killer. You're lucky you escaped."

"Luck nothing, he fought his way out," Frenchie said indignantly, "I told you he was okay."

"What would Killer want with the book," Toot asked.

"I have no idea," Godfrey said. "He's on their side?"

"Doctor X is practicing on his people, I bet he wants revenge. Diablo said someone named Gloria told him. The only Gloria I know is a housekeeper at the hospital …" Dean's voice trailed off. "She probably heard me talking. She hates me."

"That would be his cousin," Godfrey said with a half-amused smile. "Frenchie did say you've been telling everyone and his brother about the book. So, now, Doctor X knows who you are, and so does Killer. Frankly, I'd take my chances with Doctor X. Let me get this straight, you wasted those guys?"

"I guess I did," Dean answered. His mind was still reeling from what had happened. "It all happened so fast."

"Well, I have two things to say," Godfrey said. "First, you're obviously tougher than you look. And second, you better hope the world does come to an end, because Killer is gonna come after you, and he makes those guys look like choir boys."

"Or we solve this case, save the world and become heroes," Frenchie said. "Then no one will touch Dean, and maybe Killer goes to jail."

"So the two of you, the two of you, will be going up against the Doctor X gang *and* the Death Masters. One impossibility wasn't enough, was it?"

"We'll have the cops meet us there," Dean rasped, holding his sides. "I'll find a way to get them up there, I'll figure out something. But we've got to do something, sitting around is no longer an option. If this thing is on the level …"

"Can you help us, big brother?" Frenchie asked her lifelong friend.

"Do you really believe this stuff, French?" Godfrey asked. "Do you really believe in this conspiracy?"

She paused.

"I believe in Dean. Can you help us?"

Godfrey looked at Frenchie and smiled gently.

"Sure, why not," he said. "I get you up there, and I'll protect you on the way. Just remember, before the cops, or cavalry, or whatever, come, me and Toot are out of there. I'm not allowed to fight. I'm not even supposed to leave the city without checking first with my PO. We're just dropping you off. And no executions for desertion, okay?"

Dean averted his eyes, slightly embarrassed.

"I'm sorry, Dean, it just came up in our talk," Frenchie said awkwardly.

"Yeah, right," Godfrey said good-naturedly. "She almost ripped my head off."

"So, what do we do now," Toot asked.

"First, we fix the good doctor up," Godfrey replied, sounding almost businesslike. "He'll draw too much attention the way he looks now. And then we get some transportation. I'll be rooting for you guys— I don't want those kids dying either. Toot, I didn't tell anyone about Jungle Man, so it can be said that I kept my word. Toot, you coming along?"

"Sure, let's see what the gods want. But I won't, I can't, hurt any of my brothers."

"All right, everyone, listen up," Godfrey said. "It's starting to get dark. Wait here. Toot and I will be back in a few minutes."

The two men walked off.

Frenchie carefully cleaned Dean's face, worriedly frowning as she looked at his wounds. She lifted his hand to her lips and kissed it. He relaxed, and would have hugged her had his chest not hurt so much.

"I do love you," she said.

They sat together on the steps, holding hands. Dean shivered slightly in the cool early evening breeze, grateful that the air was relatively warm. After a short while he caught sight of Godfrey rounding the corner in a shiny, late model sedan. Toot sat next to him. The car pulled up in front of the building.

"Come on, honey, it's time to get the bad guys," Frenchie said.

"Where, where'd they get this car?" Dean asked incredulously.

"Come on," Frenchie said. "We'll talk later."

She helped him to his feet, and they slowly walked to the car. Frenchie opened the back door and they got in. The car sped off.

I've passed it, Dean thought, slinking down in the backseat without realizing it. I've passed the point of no return. I just killed two people, and now I'm driving through town in a stolen car, most likely with career criminals. There's a street gang after me. Frankly, if I am very, very lucky, I will have my encounter with this person Doctor X. Because either I save the world, or I'm a dead man.

chapter 52

Connigan rearranged several vials on the table. Spread out before him were many test tubes, each filled with fluid. Mr. Natural, who had just arrived, began carefully placing them in labeled metal canisters and screwing on the lids. A large beaker, having just simmered, was now being allowed to cool.

Their cabin was quiet. With no electricity or plumbing, and nothing outside but the slowly darkening forest, they felt peacefully adrift, lost in time and space. There were no fears of intrusion from the outside world; their guards were like the dark violet clouds above, silent, floating, and in their own way, completely reliable.

"Just like in the movies, huh?" Mr. Natural said, chuckling as he handled the bottles. "I never knew I'd enjoy working with a mad scientist so much."

He wasn't looking at Connigan and did not see his pained look. The guard got up and walked to the window.

"Are we done soon?" he asked, peering out at the trees. "I'll feel much better when all this is in the cave."

"Just about," the scientist replied. He stopped. "Let me ask you, what do you really want most when the change comes?"

"Brother, I want the magic to return. Everything's all machines now. It's a big wasteland out there. The essence, the spirits, the magic, everything's gone. The elves, fairies, wizards, all gone. But just temporarily, mind you. They'll come back when the time is right. And I'll be there to greet them."

"I figured you'd say something like that," Connigan mumbled, going back to his vials.

"What's so bad about that?" Mr. Natural asked defensively.

"Nothing, nothing at all."

"My one regret is that I won't get to see the faces of all the phonies who sold out and went back to their empty lives," Mr. Natural said. "I was the only one from the commune who stayed true. We used to chant together, get high together and make plans about the new world. Now they all live in condos, own digital bullshit, drink martinis, make deals and think I'm a fool. And you know what? A lot of times, when I had to scrape for rent, I did feel like a fool. Yeah, next week, before the epidemic hits, while it's still percolating, I'm gonna be making a lot of phone calls. I'm gonna say, 'Hey, man, remember when we sat by the fire, talking about nirvana and utopia? Well, baby, they're around the corner and you ain't gonna see 'em. Put that in your hard drive."

The security guard laughed heartily. When he noticed Connigan's somber look, he cleared his throat indignantly.

"And what do you want most to come back," Mr. Natural asked brusquely. "Come on, I told you, you tell me ..."

"The peace," Connigan whispered sadly.

"What was that?" Mr. Natural asked, leaning forward.

There was a gentle knock on the door. It opened, and a dark Indian respectfully entered. Behind him were three heavily armed men.

"Doctor, the time has come," one of them said slowly.

Connigan was very still.

"So it has," he finally said.

He picked up the cooled beaker and poured its clear contents into a vial layered with whitish powder. The mixture immediately turned a deep blue. Connigan smiled tightly and nodded to himself. Mr. Natural looked on in fascination. The scientist quickly sealed the vial and placed in a marked container.

"Give this to Doctor X," he said. "It is the key to everything."

Mr. Natural rose to his feet and carefully picked up the container.

Connigan looked up at him. His stare made the guard turn away uncomfortably. He pretended to look at something outside the window.

"Guess I'll be going," he finally said. "What about you?"

"Go meet your spirits," Connigan answered. "I'll wait here."

chapter 53

Killer hammered his kitchen table with his giant fist. The loud noise only increased his agitation. He raised his hand again and pounded even harder. The wooden table shattered into small pieces.

He had never been in such a fury. Diablo had raced back to the club like a crazy man. His nearly incoherent description of the two mutilated men now burned in his brain like acid. At first Killer refused to believe him. They ran back to Dean's block, but turned back when they saw police cars, lights flashing, parked in front of the building. They knew they were too late, they would never see their men again.

Killer lifted his bottle of vodka, taking several large gulps. He had drunk half by now and was waiting for the big calm, but was only feeling more anger. He felt tight and excited on the inside. It was even worse when he closed his eyes. It was as if he could see his rage, coiled and twisted before him like a giant snake. His emotions were becoming unbearable. Suddenly, he knew what he must do.

Without shutting a light, locking the door, or looking back, Killer tore out of his apartment and raced down the stairs. He ran out of his shabby building and down the street, unmindful of the stares around him. He didn't care. He kept running as fast as he could, heading downtown, five blocks, ten blocks. He was in excellent condition and barely broke a sweat. If anything, the run made him feel stronger.

Within minutes he was on Dean's block. Although less than a mile away from his neighborhood, this upscale area could have been another world. Well dressed professionals moved in every direction, radiating success. The streets were clean. Specialty stores abounded here, selling things like antiques and artwork, something unheard of where he lived. The entire place exuded an air of self-confidence, safety and exclusivity.

Killer hated being here because when he was, he felt stupid and useless, and people looked at him not with respect or admiration, but as if he were a dirty, dangerous animal. And today he despised these streets even more, because somewhere on them was the doctor who had humiliated him.

He walked up to Dean's building. The police cars were gone, but two men in uniform appeared to be posted at the front entrance. To keep out garbage like me, he thought darkly. Rage again bubbled inside him, almost bringing tears to his eyes.

I've got to do something, he thought, doubling over as if punched. Otherwise, I'll explode.

He resumed running, looking for an outlet for his boiling emotions. He knew, as he was moving, that he was going to kill someone.

Soon he saw a young couple walking up cement steps, going into a private brownstone. They were trim and elegant, each in their own way very attractive. Killer instantly selected them to die.

He slowed his pace as he approached their building, timing his moves perfectly. He watched the man laughingly fumble for his front door key, while the woman playfully tickled him under his trench coat to distract him. They were completely oblivious to his presence. Killer smiled wickedly. They don't even know that this is their last minute, he thought. Just like cattle in the yards.

As the front door heaved open Killer ran up the steps, slamming into both of them, hurling them forward into the building's carpeted hallway. He followed his sprawling victims inside and shut the door behind him.

Thirty minutes later, he casually opened the door and ambled down the street. He was wearing the dead man's watch and bracelet. All punched out and finally drained of all energy, sexual as well as physical, he felt relaxed and finally able to think clearly.

Got to do two things, he thought, lighting a cigarette, using the dead man's silver plated lighter. First, find this Doctor X, the one who's hunting my men. I don't know who he is, but I know where he's gonna be. Tonight, he's gonna pay for messing with me.

He patted the copy of Connigan's book in his pocket. Little Bear Park, he thought. I went there as a kid.

And that brings me to the second thing. I'm gonna get that Miller, the one who wasted my guys today. He's gonna get treated extra special.

Walking with an almost defiant casualness, rubbing his crotch and thinking about the woman he had just taken, he strolled down the street. As always, he reveled in the unease he inspired among passersby, and he made a point of dangling his blood stained hands prominently for all to see. Open pathways seemed to spring up before him like magic, as people scurried out of the way.

When he had reached the border area, near his neighborhood, he pulled out the dead man's cell phone and called his club. He rang once, hung up, rang twice, and hung up again. Then he called and stayed on the line, having signaled to the other side that it was a Death Master calling. He studied his new watch as the phone rang, nodding with admiration.

"Yeah?" Diablo asked.

"It's me."

"Where you been, man? Everybody's been …"

"Don't worry about it. Now do as I say. Get everyone together. I don't care if they're drinking, gambling or getting their dick licked. I want everyone ready in thirty minutes. We're fighting tonight."

"Fighting? Killer, half the guys are dead!"

"I don't think you heard me. We're fighting. You got a problem with that?"

"No, man," Diablo said contritely. "You want it, you got it."

"Tonight we fix the guy who's been hunting us. And maybe we'll even see that Doctor Miller."

"Killer, leave him for me?"

"We'll see. Remember, thirty minutes, everyone meets at the club. We're taking a little drive."

Killer put the phone away and extracted some money from the dead man's wallet. He decided to go into a nearby deli and get something to eat. It's gonna be a busy night, he thought, and all this stuff is working up an appetite.

chapter 54

The drive out of the city went smoothly. It was well past rush hour, and traffic was light. Dean stared at the slowly darkening scenery. He was trying to digest the fact he had left his phone at the apartment and none of his companions had one—a cornerstone of the plan he had been formulating had just crumbled.

"Beautiful here, isn't it?" he said aloud, trying to cheer himself up. "One of my patients moved up here recently, his sister has a farm. He invited me to visit but I never took him up on it. Now I wish I had."

A police cruiser passed them. Dean felt his insides turn icy cold. He leaned forward and politely tapped Godfrey on the shoulder.

"We are driving nice and safe, right?"

"Don't worry, Doc, it's middle lane all the way. I'm allergic to blue."

"Until later, of course. You do realize that we need the police. Right?"

"If you say so. But I'm telling you now, when they come, I go. And you never saw me before, just like I never saw you."

"You really don't mean that," Dean said. "You'll be a hero."

"And you can keep my medal, too."

Godfrey turned up the radio, effectively ending all conversation. Dean sat back in the seat, slightly frowning. Frenchie gently tapped his arm.

"Don't be hard on him, he's had it rough," she said quietly. "Aside from growing up in the worst neighborhood there ever was, he's had his share of bad luck. What makes it worse is that deep down I swear he always wanted to be a cop."

"You're kidding. He was the leader of the Death Masters."

"We were all something back then, we did what we thought we had to do. I'm telling you, Godfrey wasn't mean enough for his own gang. He didn't rob, and he never hit women. He acted badder than he was. Once in a while he'd put on a show when they fought another gang. Boy, could he kick ass."

She looked out the window, reminiscing.

"Yeah, he was something else," she whispered. "Nobody ever realized, even once, that he never hit an innocent person. That was his little secret. I even saw him cry once, although he'd call me a liar."

"What made him cry?" Dean asked, surprised.

"Some kids set his dog on fire when he left the gang. She died in his arms."

Dean shuddered. What a world, he thought.

"Godfrey should have gone to school," he finally said. "He seems very smart."

"He's damn smart. It kills me to see him mop floors. It's like watching a caged lion in some zoo."

"He'd be a good person to bring along for this little expedition," Dean said. "Brains and brawn."

"Yeah. Though you ain't no slouch yourself. You beat up a few of those Indians, and you killed two Death Masters. Godfrey won't let on, but I can tell he's impressed."

Her words, though casually spoken, had a chilling effect. I really did those things, he thought. I'm becoming as bad as the people I'm fighting.

"I didn't mean to do any of that," he blurted out. "It was pure survival. There was no pleasure involved. It was like instinct ... you know, they were going to kill me."

"Honey, it's okay."

"The first guy, I figured he'd faint if I jabbed his eyes," he continued desperately. "The sudden rise in pressure could do that, and he may not even be dead, just, uh, blind. God, what have I done? With the second man, it happened so fast. I slashed him with his own razor, the one he was going to use on me. It hit the carotid artery, the jugular, the trachea. He died for sure, probably from blood loss."

"Man, you're in this deep," Frenchie said softly.

"What do you mean," Dean asked anxiously, biting his lower lip.

"Well, if the Death Masters don't get you, and Killer must have at least twenty guys left, then the cops are going to have lots of questions. I assume your guests are still in your apartment. "

Dean covered his face with his hands.

"This whole thing is legit, right?" she asked.

"Oh, I sure hope so."

"Then don't worry about it. You're gonna be famous. They'll put your picture on stamps, money, you name it. Killer won't even think of hurting you. Hell, he'll be grateful that you saved him from the disease."

Dean looked around morosely.

"Somehow that does not cheer me up," he said.

They exited the highway and drove along a quiet road. Dean signaled for them to pull over at a small shopping center. Godfrey and Toot stayed in the car. Dean and Frenchie got out and walked into a convenience store, holding hands. When they entered the clerk and the few customers there instantly braced for a robbery. Dean was startled at their response. Do we look that scary, he asked himself, or just that different.

Trying to look casual, he purchased a few flashlights and candles, and scooped up a few candy bars. While the clerk nervously waited for his credit card to be approved, Dean could feel several stares boring into his back. He had the urge to run out of the store but resisted. Covered with bruises, but wearing obviously new but not quite matching clothes that Toot had somehow obtained, he knew that any unusual motion would result in a firestorm of attention. Stay calm, he thought, this isn't the time to be conspicuous.

Leaving the store, he could almost hear the sighs of the people inside. The car was parked around the corner, far out of view, so that no one from the store saw it, where it came from, or which direction it would be headed. Very cute, Dean thought, Godfrey gets an A in street smarts.

They drove several more miles and pulled into a gas station. Dean looked at the fuel gauge—the tank was three quarters full.

"Why are we stopping?" he asked.

"You said you wanted to call the police," Godfrey said, pointing to a pay phone. We don't have a phone, and you can't exactly ask Doctor X for his when you get there. So here's you're chance."

He nudged Toot, who was napping in the front seat.

"This is a first in my life," he said. "Me, telling someone to call in the law."

Dean and Godfrey got out of the car, and walked over to a pay phone alongside the station. The glass panels were missing, but to Dean's relief the dial tone was loud and clear.

"Are you sure you want to do this," Godfrey asked softly.

"Who should I call?" Dean asked. "The FBI? CIA?"

"Well, I don't have too much experience with those groups, having only been a petty thief myself," Godfrey answered. "Why don't you just start small and call the cops. See what they have to say."

"The local police?"

Godfrey looked around.

"It's pretty quiet around these parts. With luck you might get a deputy. I don't think they'll raise much of a posse for you."

"I guess I'll call down to the city," Dean said. "I bet they could get up here in time, or at least coordinate something with someone up here …"

"Suit yourself."

"I even know the number to the police office at the hospital. I'll let them handle it."

He dialed, fed the phone a bunch of coins, and waited.

"Lieutenant Brandt," a voice said.

"Lieutenant, this is Doctor Miller. You may or may not remember me, I don't really care. Listen and do not interrupt. A great many people are going to die. I do not have anything to do with it, but I can stop it with your help. You have got to believe me."

He saw Godfrey wince at his words.

"Talk fast, because they just started tracing the call," Godfrey said. "They'll be here in ten minutes, you can bet on it."

"You're the ER doctor, aren't you? Miller, what's going on, where are you?" the officer demanded.

"Don't talk to me like that! You should have listened to me instead of acting like a jerk," Dean shot back. He rubbed his face, which was throbbing and painful. His joints ached and he felt like he weighed a million pounds.

Godfrey leaned over and whispered in his ear.

"Be cool, Doc, let's do the job and wrap it up," he counseled.

Dean nodded, feeling slightly foolish. God, it's so hard staying focused, he thought.

"Lieutenant, I'm sorry. Look, there's some group that's going to unleash some kind of germ warfare bomb. Tonight. It will cause unbelievable destruction."

Dean could hear muffled sounds at the other end of the line.

"Talk very fast," Godfrey said, rolling his eyes upward.

"Go to Little Bear Park," Dean continued rapidly. "I'll meet you at the main entrance. I know where they're hiding. We'll get them together."

"You're the doctor who lives on 74th Street, right?"

"Yes, that's me," Dean said, perplexed. He had not been expecting this reply.

"Doctor, we've been looking for you. You're needed for questioning, it's pretty important. We can talk about this park thing at the same time. Where are you?"

"You've been looking for me?" Dean stammered. "What type of questioning?"

Then he remembered the two bodies in his apartment. His jaw dropped and he stood there, as if frozen.

"I'm going back to the car," Godfrey warned. "I'm serious, be back in one minute."

"Nothing to worry about, Doc," the policeman continued. "We'll discuss everything when you come in."

His tone had changed from irritable to businesslike, with a touch of phony sweetness, and he seemed to talk more slowly now, as if playing for time.

"If you prefer, Doctor Miller, if it's a bother, we can pick you up and personally drive you in. It's no hassle for us. Where's your location?"

"Look, I can't talk. Meet me in about an hour at Little Bear Park. Main entrance. Okay? Gotta go."

"Doctor!"

Dean slammed the receiver down. At that moment Godfrey honked the car horn impatiently. Waving to him, Dean ran over and got in. The car sped off. To everyone's relief the road remained quiet.

Godfrey drove through the small town, makings several turns. When he was convinced they weren't being followed, he pulled over at a near empty truck stop. For a few moments no one spoke. Frenchie bit her lip and stared out the rear window. Toot stretched lazily in the front seat.

"That was horrible," Dean exclaimed. "I actually got the impression of being a wanted criminal."

"It does sound like it," Godfrey said quietly, looking around, slightly nervous. "I didn't realize they'd be on to you so quick. Then again, it is a double homicide."

"On to me," Dean stammered. He thought of the razor he had left at the apartment. "That wasn't murder."

"Of course not," Godfrey said distractedly, looking around. "Please talk lower, okay?"

"He did not commit murder," Frenchie echoed, squeezing Dean's hand.

"Then you'll get off, Doc. They'll see your bruises, you say they tried to rob you, and plead self defense. They'll go for it, you're a doctor, and those guys you wasted have rap sheets bigger than a phone book. Thank goodness it wasn't me. I'd be making license plates by the weekend."

"That cop didn't believe me."

"Probably not," Godfrey said, easing the car back onto the highway. "But they will. What're you going to do now?"

"Do you think the police will help us find Doctor X?" Dean asked weakly.

"You mean, send a SWAT team into the woods, with you leading the charge? Probably not. That little plan of yours crashed and burned. Right now they just want to take you in. Maybe they'll sniff around the place tomorrow, but it will be too late by then, won't it?"

Godfrey shook his head sadly. Then he looked up at Dean.

"Do you still want to go for it? Then drive up to the park, ditch the car, and avoid the main entrance. Go on and fight your battle. Toot and I, we'll figure a way to get home. Or, do you want to call it a day and go back home?"

"I'm not giving up now, I can't and I won't!" Dean said, slamming a fist into his hand. "There are fanatics out there trying to kill us. And they will if I don't stop them. *Me*, of all people. I'm not the hero type, Godfrey, I didn't ask for this job. But no, I am not going home."

"Then it's time to come up with plan B, Doc."

Dean stared out the window. It can't be hopeless, he thought. It's like one of Frenchie's puzzles, it's just a giant maze, and this is just one of the dead ends. There is a way out of this.

Frenchie sympathetically caressed Dean's face. Godfrey stared at them through the rear view mirror. Toot slept quietly in the front seat.

Suddenly Dean sat upright, he face taut with determination.

"Godfrey, pull over to the next pay phone you see," he said, his voice full of authority.

"You got it, boss," Godfrey said, a smile on his face.

They stopped at another gas station. This time Dean got out alone. He walked over to the phone, dialed information, wrote down a number, and dialed once more. Elated that his party was home, he spoke animatedly. His companions watching him in amazement as he spoke.

Back in the car Frenchie tried to read his lips.

"Who is he talking to?" she asked aloud.

"Beats me," Godfrey said. "He seems to be giving out directions. He's an interesting guy. And you know what, the man's okay. Frenchie, I officially approve."

"Why, thank you, big brother," she said, smiling. "I bet we can make a go of it."

"Listen, the big thing in life is finding the one person you want to share it with. I'm really glad for you, I think you're going to do okay with this guy."

"I'll be good to him."

"I know you will, French."

Dean walked back to the car. He seemed more confident.

"It's time to meet Doctor X," he said. "No cops, I just took care of them."

"You did, huh?" Godfrey said, amused.

"Yes. I'll drive the car. If we do get stopped I take the blame for everything, even the car. You just came along for the ride. Toot, keep me company."

Godfrey thought for a moment, and then got out. He stretched his large frame, and then looked down at Dean. Without a word, he got into the back seat.

Seconds later they were heading straight for Little Bear Park.

chapter 55

The trip was progressing smoothly and actually had a soothing effect on Dean, whose pains gradually started to ebb. Traffic was light on this weekday night. Dean drove carefully, the cruise control set exactly at the legal speed limit.

No one spoke, Toot had his eyes half closed. Godfrey and Frenchie seemed to be asleep in the back seat, their heads leaning against each other. After a while, Dean found the silence unbearable. He couldn't get over how relaxed Toot was, how unperturbed he seemed to be by all of the recent events.

"Rough stuff going on, huh?" he said, trying to make some talk.

"I guess," Toot replied absently, looking out the window.

"Do you think we'll find Doctor X?"

"Of course, Doc, you're pretty smart."

"You've been so quiet, Toot, is anything wrong?"

"I've been thinking about home."

"The city?"

"The jungle. Where I grew up is a spice plantation now. I wish they had left it alone—they had no right to do that. We were on that land for a thousand years. I was thinking how I'd like to go back. Sometimes when I'm in the subway I close my eyes and make believe that if I stay on until the last stop, boom, I'm back in the forest."

"You really want to go back?"

"Yeah. Jungle Man says we're all going back."

"Jungle Man. Toot, I know he's your friend, but listen, please—he's doing something that can possibly hurt a great many people. That's why I have to stop him. To prevent a lot of suffering. There are better ways to save the world."

"He's a good man, Doc."

"I'm not saying he's not."

"Our people believe that only good people join their ancestors when they die. Everyone else rots in the ground and their spirit disappears. He would never make his people do anything bad, he loves them too much. And I love him like my father. When I came to the city he took me in. I was eating garbage back then, and living on the streets."

"Incredible. When was that?" Dean asked, trying to change the subject, not wanting to possibly antagonize his companion.

"I have no idea, Doc. Back then I didn't know the day, month or year. I just lived. That's what I liked about the jungle. You didn't need this stuff. I don't read or write, and I only know a few numbers. I won't need them when I go back, so I'm glad I didn't waste the time."

Dean felt lost in Toot's presence. In some ways we have a lot in common, he thought, but sometimes it's like we're two different species. It's funny, I have this urge to convert him into me, probably because I don't understand him. I wonder if he'd like to change me.

He decided to change the subject one more time. Now is not exactly the time to compare cultural values, he thought. After we save this crazy world, we'll co-sponsor a conference or something.

"So, the jungle's dangerous?"

"If you don't know what you're doing. The pigs are the scariest. Up here, pigs are funny, but down there, they're the most dangerous of all the animals. Except for the snakes, maybe, which hang from the branches. Man, you can walk right into them if you're not careful. But the pigs, they're big and nasty. They travel in packs, and they attack you if they catch you alone. They start eating you once you fall to the ground. They don't bother killing you first. We were more afraid of them than the big cats."

Toot shook his head, reminiscing.

"I remember when they chased me and my friend. I got away. My friend, he climbed a tree, and sat right on this giant snake. It killed him right off. We went back and got him a few days later. I still dream about it. My friend had turned black."

"Why was he all black," Dean asked, grimacing.

"The heat. When you die, it melts your fat and turns black. Then it drips out of your skin. It looks like you were wiped up and down with grease. You get all shiny and ..."

"Sounds just great," Dean said, looking at the exits. "So are there snakes and pigs all over the jungle. Even where you sleep?"

"No, it's cool. Doc, you'd love it there. It's the center of the world, did you know that?"

"With my luck, I'd get lost in five minutes, and a few days later, they'd find me, all black and ..."

"Don't worry, Doc. If you get lost I'd come and get you. Just like you got me."

Dean smiled. Toot remembered, after all. Four years ago, on a frozen winter's night, he had come wandering in, clearly under the influence of some hallucinogen. He was acting crazed and confused, and on the stretcher he became very agitated. Ripping out all his tubes, and wearing only a paper thin gown, he had run out of the ER, bleeding from two IV sites.

Most of the ER staff just laughed, and a sneering ward clerk picked up the phone to contact the police.

"Well, we're gonna have a *'shpos-cicle,'*" one of the doctors quipped.

While they were placing bets on how low Toot's body temperature was going to be when the police found him, Dean jumped from his chair and ran out of the ER.

"Dean, where you going?" one of his colleagues called out.

"To find him," he called out.

"You're as crazy as he is," Molloy shouted. "If the snowdrifts won't get you, the muggers will. Don't leave the fort."

Dean remembered how he had wandered through the dark snow, shivering with cold in his flimsy lab coat, his sneakers filled with icy slush. He remembered how dark and barren the streets looked in the dead of the night, these same streets that pulsed frenetically during the day. The dark seemed to absorb all light, and the snow all sound; it felt as if he were traveling in a lost world.

Finally, he found Toot, who had collapsed under a parked car. Picking up the naked man, he carried him in his arms, stumbling but never falling, unmindful of his burning arms or frozen toes, back to the ER. Nine days later, after an initial stormy course which was touch and go, Toot was discharged. He walked through the ER to thank everyone, and to drop off a bag of homemade cookies. Before he left, he looked at Dean.

"I'll never forget you," he had said.

"Don't mention it," Dean replied awkwardly, mindful of the stares of his colleagues.

After Toot shuffled out, using a cane, Finkel spoke up.

"Dean, I've got to say, he does seem almost human. After factoring out his drug use and those ridiculous tattoos, we're going to award you a three-quarter save, which is perhaps the highest anyone can get around here. By the way, shall we place these cookies in the circular file, or have you totally lost your mind."

"No, I have not lost my mind." There was a hint of sadness in his voice.

"Good."

With that, Finkel took the bag and threw it away. It was an unwritten rule among the staff to never, ever, eat anything from a patient that was not store bought. A few minutes later, when no one was looking, Dean stuck his hand in the garbage can and retrieved some cookies. You're very welcome, Toot, he had thought, thank you very much.

Dean came out of his reverie and looked at Toot.

"I never told you before, Toot, but the cookies were delicious."

"Gee, they told me you threw them away after I walked out."

Dean felt ashamed. How the hell did he find out, he asked himself.

"I tried them," he said awkwardly. "The others didn't know you and were afraid."

"I understand. But I'm glad you had one."

"Where'd you get them?"

"Frenchie. You're gonna like it with her, Doc. She's a great cook."

"You know, Toot, I bet I will," Dean replied, smiling. "I know I will."

chapter 56

Police Detective Peter Hawkins shoved three sticks of gum in his mouth and angrily threw the wrappers on the ground. He made a face at the shadowy woods surrounding him and swatted his neck. When he saw the bloody insect on his hand, he spat in fury.

"I should have been home by now," he snarled. "To think they'd send me to Little Bear Park. Me, with sixteen years on the force. They can keep their goddamn overtime."

"Relax, Pete, it'll be over soon," his partner, Joe Burgess said. "The city boys asked us to wait until nine. After that, they'll consider it a crank call and stand down. Who knows, the doc just may show."

"If he gives me any lip, I'll kick his goddamn ass. Leading me on a goddamn wild goose chase in the middle of the goddamn night."

"Remember, he's not under arrest. They want him for questioning."

"He's guilty as sin. You know it and I know it. And they know it. Otherwise they wouldn't have called and begged us to pick him up. They usually treat us like hicks. Until, of course, they need a favor. Like I said, if he gives me any lip …"

"Maybe you're right, but don't help some wiseass lawyer find a way to make him walk."

"Don't worry about me," Pete said. "I'll find a way to make him resist arrest. I'm too old and too smart to make a rookie mistake."

"Too old, too smart and too fat."

"Hey, at least I quit smoking. What more do you want out of my life?"

Suddenly, Joe looked into the darkness, instantly alert.

"Did you hear that?" he whispered.

"What? I didn't ..."

This time they both heard the sound, and they snapped out of their boredom, reverting to being the professionals that they were.

"It was from over there," Joe whispered, crouching behind a large bush.

They saw a solitary figure slowly walking towards them.

"I'm alerting the other car," Pete whispered back, one hand resting on his gun.

He pulled out a small transmitter.

"Bravo, do you read?"

"Bravo here. What's up?"

"We have our man. He's walking right toward us. He doesn't look armed."

"You sure it's him?"

"It's the middle of the goddamn night, in the middle of a goddamn park, fifty miles from the nearest goddamn town, and you ask if it's our man," Pete snapped. "Yes, I'm sure. But to show how nice I am, I'm even going to ask him."

"You're so sweet," the voice cackled over the speaker. "You need us up there?"

"Just stand by. We'll take him and wrap this thing up."

The two detectives crouched from their hiding point, watching the figure approach. Quickly, each sized him up, thankful for the bright moonlight. They estimated him to be of medium height and build and not overly menacing in nature. From instinct, each knew that this would not be a difficult apprehension.

"Joe, back me up," Pete said. "I'll say hello."

"Be careful," his partner said, withdrawing his gun from the holster.

The two men nodded at each other. They had been together for eight years and knew each other's thoughts and movements intimately. After countless assignments, they worked with perfect timing and coordination.

When the man was fifteen feet away, he stopped and looked around, as if listening for something. At that moment Pete stepped forward. The man visibly flinched when he saw the policeman.

"Evening, sir, can I help you?" the officer called out, holding his badge up and in front of him.

"I'm Dean Miller. Who are you?"

"Sorry, didn't mean to scare you," the officer said, carefully moving forward. "I'm Detective Hawkins. You called the police and told them to meet you here. Well, here we are. How about coming along with us?"

"Am I under arrest?"

"Do you see any handcuffs? No, all we have to do is take you in for questioning. You understand that, don't you?"

"Is this about the bodies in my apartment?"

Pete turned and looked in the direction of his partner, smiling broadly.

"Come on out, Joe, we got him."

He turned back to the man, who was shuffling nervously. Joe walked up, talking into a transmitter, not taking his eyes off the man.

"Yeah, I guess it is about the bodies," Pete said. "Just come along quietly, will you?"

"They attacked me, they broke into my apartment. You do realize it was self defense, don't you?"

The two detectives looked at each other, then at their suspect, and shrugged.

"When they find out you're a doctor, they assume you have drugs or something. I mean, do I look like I associate with gangsters?"

"I can't say that you do," Pete said, trying to size up his suspect. . "But it ain't for me to say. Come on, Doc, while I still have some blood left. These goddamn mosquitoes ..."

"Excuse me, Doctor, but what about this plot you mentioned over the phone?" Joe said. "Can you tell us something about that?"

"Sorry, I made it all up. I've been going through so much hell ..."

"Right, right, of course. Dean, you do know that falsely reporting a crime is a misdemeanor. It wasn't very smart doing that."

"I panicked, and took a cab here to hide out. I was afraid the gang was coming after me, and I wanted to make sure police would find me first. I guess I was pretty stupid."

"I'll say," Pete said with disgust, looking around. He wrinkled his nose and leaned forward. "You're also plastered. You a drinking man, Doc?"

"I like my beer. Listen, if you went through what I went through ..."

"Tell it to the judge." Joe said icily. "What's in that bag you're holding?"

"A sleeping bag, some supplies ..."

"C'mon, Doc, let's go."

They walked their man into the police car that had silently glided into the parking lot. All three got into the back seat, Pete and Joe on each side of their suspect. As the car pulled away, its lights flashing, each gave the other a thumb's up sign.

"Call the city boys," Pete told the driver, scratching a mosquito bite on his arm. "Tell them to meet us at the county line. And tell them they owe us. I don't think I have one drop of blood left."

When they were several miles away from the state park, heading south for the city, Bob McElvoy finally relaxed in the back seat. His bones ached from the cancer spreading through them, but he was happy. I ran a good tackle for you, Doctor Miller. I don't know what it was for, but I ran a good tackle. I'm glad you called and asked for the favor. Good luck, whatever you're going to do up there.

He leaned back in the seat, trying to wish away the pain, half wishing he had actually drunk the beer he had poured over himself. He stole a look at the burly policemen on each side of him and secretly smiled. I should have gone into acting, he thought. And I can't blame the doctor for not wanting these guys around, they're definitely uncouth.

The police car, with escorts in front of and behind it, raced through the night, heading for the city line.

chapter 57

The trip had gone smoothly. At one point five cars, racing at top speed, shot past them, vanishing into the distance. There was another tense moment a few minutes later, when three police cars headed towards them, their lights flashing. Everyone held their breath. But they kept going and again nothing happened. Minutes later they approached the entrance to Little Bear State Forest.

When he was sure that there were no other police cars around, Dean quickly turned inside and cut off his lights. He drove into a parking area he remembered from previous trips, grimly taking note of the many cars and two large vans already there. Granted, it's a hot night, he thought, but it's still May, way too early for the overnight crowd. It looks like Doctor X just may be out there somewhere.

This was a huge state park, nearly three hundred thousand acres in size. Through popular by day, at night it was usually empty until the summer camping season. After having been in the city for so long, he was struck by its vast, imposing openness. In the night air, it transmitted a sense of mysterious grandeur.

They parked as far as they could from the other vehicles and got out, each holding a flashlight and a small bag of supplies. It took a few seconds for their eyes to become accustomed to the silvery moonlight, which bathed the entire area with a ghostly radiance. Dean forgot how well one could see by a full moon; though colors ceased to exist, one could see with a strange, almost exciting, clarity not possible during the day.

He walked a few feet from the car, looking around. Frenchie approached him from behind.

"Do you still love me?" she asked quietly. "You don't have to keep all those promises you made back there if you don't want to, I'd understand."

Dean kissed her.

"I'm with you all the way. And you're with me, right?"

"All the way."

Holding her hand, he walked back to the car. Godfrey and Toot were waiting patiently.

"Are you guys going back?" Dean asked. "Godfrey, the cavalry was sent back home, it's just us and the bad guys. Can you help me? If you can't, I'll understand, and there won't be any hard feelings."

Godfrey breathed deeply.

"Air's nice around here. Yeah, I'll do what I can. I've been thinking, no one has the right to do this. Not you, not me, not them. And who knows, maybe this will atone for some of the bad stuff I did when I was younger."

"Toot?" Dean asked, looking at the smaller man, who seemed to be frowning.

"Jungle Man is with this Doctor X?" he finally asked.

"Yes, of course," Dean said. "Remember those people in the courtyard, and the ones in the hospital? That was Doctor X testing out the sickness. Jungle Man was helping him, he captured those men for the experiment. He's one of them, Toot, don't you know that?"

"Yeah, I guess. Doc, I'm having trouble with this. You saved my life, and you're trying to save your world, but Jungle Man, he's like my father, and he's trying to save his world. I love all of you, but deep down I'm one of them. You world has the power , but I swear it doesn't have the spirit. It has no honor or respect.

"I won't stop you, I won't hurt you, but I can't help you. If the gods want you to stop Doctor X, then you will."

Dean nodded his understanding. He had secretly wondered how long Toot would last, and he wasn't surprised at his words.

"Wait here by the car," he said quietly. "Here are my keys and my watch. If we're not back in four hours then you drive out of here. You can drive, can't you?"

"If it's okay with you guys, let me tag along. You have my word that I won't get in the way. I have to see how this thing ends. It's just that I feel sort of trapped between sides, know what I mean?"

Dean looked at Godfrey, who nodded, yes, you can trust him.

"Sure, Toot, come on," Dean said. "What's a war without a conscientious objector?"

Before handing over his watch to Toot he stole a glance at it.

"If the book is right, we have two hours. It may get pretty wild, and I'm not really sure what to do when we get there, except maybe to knock over chemicals, pour out the test tubes, you know, things like that. And it's going to be dangerous. This operation is too sophisticated not to be guarded. Surprise is probably our only advantage. So please, use the lights only if necessary. Okay everyone, ready?"

They all nodded.

With Dean leading the way, they walked in single file along the grassy path. The moonlight was more than adequate in this relatively open area. No one spoke, and they instinctively walked low to the ground. In the back of everyone's mind was the fact that somewhere in this forest was Doctor X. Soon enough, if all went as planned, the unplanned would shortly be the norm.

After a few hundred yards the path turned into the forest itself, and suddenly and irrevocably, they were enveloped by the trees. The clearing and parking lot, and all signs of civilization, completely vanished from their sights, and within seconds, from their minds.

Dean stopped and motioned for a conference. They huddled around him.

"The campsite is about a mile from here. I've been there twice. We have to go up this path and look for a blue diamond sign. Then we take that trail until we get there. The trees are marked with blue plastic dots so you can't get lost."

"I'm lost already," Frenchie said, looking around.

"What exactly do we do when we get to this place?" Godfrey asked.

"I don't know—make some noise to distract them, to decoy them into the forest. Then I'll run up and destroy their equipment."

"An intricate plan, indeed," Godfrey said, "I just hope you don't get shot or something."

Dean paused. I could easily get killed tonight, he thought.

"Godfrey, do you have any weapons?" he asked.

"I could throw the flashlight at them."

"Well, we'll worry about that later. The point is, our families, friends, everyone, will all die if we fail. This is for real. I know my plan is flawed, but unless someone comes up with something better, it's all we have. So, let's hit the road."

They resumed walking down the path. It was darker here because of the surrounding foliage, and they concentrated on the ground, using their flashlights to light their way. The forest was eerily silent and appeared speckled all around them with silvery light; everything beyond several yards was remote and shadowy.

Dean cursed his feet for the crunching sound they made in the stillness and was astounded that Toot walked in near silence.

"How do you walk so quietly?" he whispered in frustration to Toot.

"I don't know, Doc, how do you read X-rays?"

At times, while they trudged along the narrow path, Dean felt the dark woods closing in on him. He fought back his fear. It's nonsense, he thought. A few hours ago this place was green and playful. Just because the sun goes down it doesn't mean evil spirits and monsters come out. And obviously there are no dangerous animals, at least not any more. At least not any on four legs, a small voice within him said.

Still, he couldn't get over his feelings that these woods were somehow possessed of an ancient wildness, and that the trappings of civilization had retreated into the distant towns many miles away. He felt lost, a city boy in the midst of the primal elements, and realized how hopelessly out of touch he was with nature.

He turned to look back at his companions. Godfrey was behind him, moving with a graceful power. After him was Toot, who appeared positively serene, almost floating as he walked, his jungle prowess clearly coming back to him. He's so wasted in the city, Dean thought, he's a prince out here.

At the rear was Frenchie, who was struggling over twigs and rocks, her teeth clenched. At one point she stumbled and nearly fell. Dean caught his breath as he watched her trip. Toot noticed Dean's reaction, and he too looked back. Effortlessly he seemed to glide back on the path and in a second was with her. With an almost touching graciousness, he extended his arm, as if to escort her onto a ballroom floor. She gratefully accepted it, and they began walking together, arm in arm, each smiling. Dean turned back and resumed walking towards the campsite.

They made slow but steady progress, going deeper and deeper into the forest. This section was meant for serious hikers, and there was no trace of the outside world. The trail they were on intersected and forked with several others, each looking the same. In the darkness Dean prayed that he was taking them the correct way. If they were lost they wouldn't be able to find their way out until daylight.

His mind drifted as he walked, the totally alien scene loosening his grip on time and place. He imagined countless men before him, for hundreds of thousands of years, walking through woods identical to these, under the light of this same moon. Hell, I could be anywhere now, and this could be anytime, he thought. I'd forgotten how basic it all really is.

He recalled a night walk he took with his father many years ago on a scouting trip. It's like yesterday, he thought. God, it even looks and smells the same. He remembered how he had walked alongside his father—he felt that the world was perfect and that all things were taken care of. He remembered how they made barking and yipping noises as they went along, laughing all the while, each trying to top the other. The louder or funnier the sound, the louder they would laugh. Dean remembered how the tears rolled down his face. He was so happy. When his father noticed, he had picked him up and kissed him. Every time Dean would stumble on a branch or rock, his father was there to hold him steady. One image kept coming back. Under the moonlight, while they were crossing a tiny stream, he looked up and said, "I love you, Dad." He hugged his father and kissed him on his belly. And then his father had started crying.

A week later. Dean walked into his kitchen to get a bowl of cereal and saw his mother sitting at the table, with a strange look in her eyes.

"Dad moved out," she said.

So many lifetimes ago, Dean thought, his skin tingling. In a lot of ways I stopped growing after that day. I certainly stopped loving. Why did you do it, Dad, why did you leave me? Why did you let the center of me die like that? Why?

Under the moon's glow, in the midst of the dark forest, Dean began to cry, as he prayed that, at that moment, somehow, his father would come back, and that they could continue their walk, and hold hands once again.

There was a tap on his shoulder, and he stared violently, whirling around. Godfrey jumped back, surprised at his response.

"You okay?" he asked cautiously.

"Yeah, sure, something got in my eye. I think it was a branch."

"You got to be careful around here," Godfrey agreed. Dean sensed the larger man knew it wasn't a branch.

The path widened at this point, and the two men walked together. Dean put away all of his old thoughts and memories. This isn't the time to deal with them, he thought to himself. Not that I ever could, but now certainly isn't the time.

"Godfrey?" he whispered.

"Yeah?"

"Why'd you leave us alone in that building?"

"There were five guys with bows and arrows aiming right at us. You didn't see them. They were in windows behind you. It was certain death to fight back. I was just playing the odds. Anyway, Toot's been speaking about Jungle Man for years, I figured he was honorable. Sorry you misunderstood."

"Yeah, all right. Another question—you were really a Death Master?"

"That was a long time ago."

"You and this person Killer were leaders?"

"Yup. But back then there were no silly names. I was Godfrey and he was, well, his name was Moses. I think that's why he started the nicknames."

"It's a tough gang, huh?"

"I think we were tougher back then. They're meaner now, and they use guns. Fighting man to man, with your hands, is almost like a lost art. We were respected, and we helped and respected each other. We were family. It's different now, it's more about drugs and money. The guys are younger and sneakier, and they have no honor. But yeah, they're bad. I wouldn't want to cross them."

"You mean like I did?"

"I would say that killing two of them constitutes crossing them."

"Is there anything I can do?" Dean asked.

"You mean, like saying you're sorry? Don't worry, if they catch you, they'll make you say it a thousand times before you die."

"You know, they were going to kill me," Dean said defensively. "They beat me, and left me lying on the floor, and one of them was coming back for more. I fought back. Is that a crime?"

"To them it is. They don't think like we do. They have no right and wrong. They're like kids in a lot of ways. And it never, ever, occurred to them that you had the right to fight back. You were supposed to die. They're outraged at what you did, and, yes, you better believe they're out for revenge."

"It's just not right."

"No, it's not. But they are all warped people, born into the wrong time and place. They could have been doctors or teachers, except that their mothers were fifteen year old dropouts who didn't have a clue. You would have become a Death Master if you were in their situation. If you made it that far. You and your colleagues, you'd all have been Death Masters."

"You may be right."

"I know I'm right."

"Are you still involved with any of them?"

"I still talk to them now and then. We'll have a beer. I mean, we still live in the same neighborhood. But most of the guys I ran with are dead or in jail. And besides, they find me pretty boring now. I don't hurt anyone anymore. I don't steal. I try to be a good person. It's been like that for a long time."

"Why did you change?"

"I started believing in God."

The path narrowed, and they resumed walking in single file.

chapter 58

Deep inside the underground cavern, Connigan poured clear liquid into a beaker, measured it carefully and added it to the large vat. As expected, the new mixture smoked gently, as one more step into the procedure was accomplished. Mr. Natural, who was standing nearby, applauded quietly. He looked across the chamber at a shrouded figure, sitting on what appeared to be a formation of rock shaped like a throne, and gave the thumb's up sign.

"I feel like one of those medieval witches," Connigan said. "With their bubbling cauldrons ..."

"Who were not inherently evil, but perceived to be so by the powers of the day," Mr. Natural interrupted. "Thus they were persecuted, as were all those who opposed the new order of cold science, intolerant religion and heartless logic."

Connigan went back to the mixture, frowning at the pain that was starting to pound inside his head.

"I happen to be a scientist, you know," he said sullenly.

Mr. Natural ignored him. He was staring at the impassive figure of Doctor X, who watched the proceedings from above them, hidden amidst the shadows and the flickering light of the fiery torches. Then he looked down at the mixture and laughed.

"To think that the Final Crusade has literally boiled down to this organic chicken soup," he said. "How appropriate that the organic womb, from which life emerged one billion years ago, has come to the rescue."

"With a little help from mankind," Connigan replied defensively. "I'm done here. The final step is all yours, and it will be ready fairly soon. You all know what to do. I'm going back to the cabin."

"And most beautifully, all other life forms will remain intact," Mr. Natural continued, half to himself. "Goodness, what are the rats and roaches going to do without all us dirty humans."

He paused as an Indian, dressed only in a loincloth, padded silently into the room. He nodded respectfully to Doctor X, and then walked up to Mr. Natural and whispered into his ear. The two conferred briefly.

"Interesting, very interesting," Mr. Natural said, smiling tightly. "The woods are rife with advancing war parties. We figured on Doctor Miller and his motley crew—he's a smart cookie. But now, now there are others … no, no no. Totally unacceptable. Professor, this is going to get interesting. Time is definitely of the essence now."

He turned to the Indian, assuming a more formal tone, and spoke to him quietly. The Indian nodded intently. Connigan craned his ear to listen, but soon gave up. He rubbed his temples dejectedly.

The Indian quickly exited, and both men turned back to the boiling mixture.

"Yes, it's going to be a most unusual evening," Mr. Natural said, as he watched the scientist turn and slowly walk away. "Most unusual indeed."

chapter 59

Dean felt a tap on his shoulder and spun around half expecting to be attacked. He had been thinking of a mountain hike in Europe many years ago and had practically forgotten why they were there.

"What is it?" he whispered, secretly disappointed to be back in these woods.

Godfrey put a finger to his lips. Shh, be quiet, he signaled. Toot and Frenchie, who were ten yards behind, had already stopped.

Godfrey pointed towards something. Dean turned, scanning the trees. When he saw the shadow, his insides twisted. A large figure was walking along an adjacent path, struggling with a large sack. Dean could hear him grunting with the weight, and for a moment the moonlight illuminated a dark face glistening with sweat. This obviously was not a camper on a nature walk, and judging from the muffled clanging sounds in the large sack, there was nothing routine about this trip.

Their paths seemed to be converging further down. Had Godfrey not noticed, they would have crossed first, and they would have been the ones discovered. Now, the advantage was theirs.

Godfrey motioned for everyone to be still, and then he went into a crouch. Silently he edged around the doctor and moved further up the trail. When he was about ten feet away from the merge point he froze, coiled and ready to spring. The whole thing was done in complete silence. Dean marveled at the man's grace.

The next few seconds lasted forever, as if the stranger was walking in slow motion and Godfrey had become a statue, waiting for him. The only noise seemed to be Dean's breathing. It was raspy and harsh, and the more he thought about it the harder it was for him to control. Fear was rising within him, and he felt it churning inside. His hands and feet began to grow numb and weak, and the sensation crept toward his center, rippling through his groin and abdomen, and then into his chest. It creeped into his neck and wrapped around it. Can't breathe, he thought in a panic, his eyes bulging, I can't breathe.

Dean struggled with all his might to stay still, but his breathing became more and more labored, his hands moving to his mouth. I'm going to suffocate, he thought madly. I can't, I can't ..."

With a roar Godfrey leaped, rushing with a speed that went faster than Dean's thoughts—he vaguely perceived the motion and the nearly instantaneous crash of the two men. For a millisecond he empathized with Godfrey's prey, sensing an awesome display of power. It wasn't until the man had been knocked down and rolled over did he actually register what had happened.

Dean ran over, suddenly aware that his anxiety attack had disappeared as quickly as it had arrived.

Godfrey knelt over his victim, twisting one of his wrists, eliciting grunts of pain. Toot and Frenchie joined them and looked down at the fallen man.

"He's all yours, Doc," he said, with a strange intensity. "It was sort of fun."

"Good work," Dean said, forcing a look of bravado. Then he gave up and put on his regular face. I'll never be a tough guy, he thought.

The man on the ground said nothing. He breathed heavily, face down, in the dirt. Suddenly he stopped struggling and lay still.

"Godfrey, frisk him."

"Already did. He's clean."

"We have to speak to him," Dean said quietly. "You think there's a chance he'll try something?"

Godfrey laughed.

"I wish he would," he replied.

"Okay, then, let's have a talk," Dean ordered.

Godfrey smiled and looked at his prisoner. He twisted a wrist; the man grunted again.

"Now behave yourself," Godfrey warned. He flipped the man over.

Dean beamed his flashlight into the man's face. His eyes bulged with surprise.

"Doctor Tannenbaum!" he whispered.

"You know this man?" Godfrey asked in bewilderment, Toot and Frenchie stared at Dean, who appeared stunned.

"Is he Doctor X?" Frenchie asked.

Dean thought of their hospital conversations and of how he had given the man Connigan's book.

"Maybe," he finally murmured, shaking his head.

"Hey, buddy, you the bad guy?' Godfrey asked his prisoner, who was squinting from the flashlight beams all directed into his face.

The man said nothing. Godfrey grabbed him tightly by the collar and pulled his face up to his.

"Are you Doctor X?" he growled.

"No, I'm Doctor Y," Tannenbaum shot back. "Doctor X couldn't make it tonight."

Godfrey was still for a moment, and then with the back of his hand smashed Tannenbaum in the face. The older man winced in pain. Dean remained silent, but inwardly was shocked at the sight of seeing his chief treated like this.

Godfrey grabbed Tannenbaum's collar and squeezed, partially choking the man.

The older doctor looked up at his assailants, blood trickling from his mouth. When he saw Dean, a shock of recognition spread over his face, followed quickly by cold hostility.

"Miller, fancy seeing you here. What is this, amateur night?"

"Answer his question."

"I'm not going to. Just let me go and you can continue making asses of yourselves. Or if you want, you can just beat me to death."

Godfrey raised his hand to strike, but Dean stopped him.

"Hold it, there's no advantage to hitting him."

"Okay for now, but I want answers," Godfrey growled, lowering his fist.

"Thanks, Miller, for calling off your dog," Tannenbaum said sarcastically. With a sudden shrug he shook free of Godfrey's grip, and sat up. "Now, get those flashlights out of my face."

Godfrey moved forward, but Dean restrained him. He signaled the others to lower their lights, which they reluctantly did. Dean hadn't figured on conducting an interrogation and tried to think of questions to ask.

"So we caught you," he finally said.

"So you did."

"I wouldn't have guessed that you were Doctor X," Dean said. "I didn't think it was possible."

"Miller, stop with the small talk. You're in over your head. My advice is to take your little pack of cub scouts back home now and stay there."

Dean was at a loss for words. He'd always admired and respected his chief, and part of him cringed with the rebuke. He struggled to find something to say.

Godfrey unwittingly intervened on his behalf. He smacked his prisoner several times in the face, slowly but powerfully, more to cause humiliation than pain. Then he violently pushed Tannenbaum backwards in the dirt. When he raised his hand as if to strike again, Tannenbaum ~~actually cringed~~ visibly flinched.

"I can do this forever," Godfrey snarled. "Answer our boss, and show some respect."

Dean looked gratefully at Godfrey, feeling stronger.

"What are you doing here?" he asked Tannenbaum.

"Just taking a nature hike."

"With that heavy bag you're carrying?" Frenchie broke in, pointing to the sack that lay several feet away. "What's in it?"

"Sugar, spice, and everything nice. I'm going to bake some muffins, Sweetie."

Frenchie appeared flustered, and looked away in embarrassment.

"Godfrey, let him go," Dean said.

The big man complied, backing away. At that exact moment Dean kicked his chief in the face. The older man rolled over in the dirt. In a moment Dean was beside him. The others watched with a mixture of fear and fascination.

"Don't ever talk to her like that," Dean hissed. "Now, give us some answers or I'll personally beat the crap out of you."

Tannenbaum seemed to crumble before them, and he became visibly subdued. "I'm too old for this. What do you want me to say?"

"What are you doing here?"

The bushes around them made a gentle rustling sound. They all briefly looked up.

"Miller, take me to the campsite," Tannenbaum finally said.

"Why, so you can wrap up the Final Crusade? Somehow that wasn't on my agenda."

"You have it so wrong."

"Then why are you here?" Dean repeated, trying not to betray his unease. This had been far too easy. The leader of a sophisticated conspiracy would never be walking alone in the forest on the night of operations.

"The same reason that you're here," Tannenbaum implored. "Only you're wasting precious time. Please, you must let me go."

"Let me worry about that," Dean replied. "How about a little talk …"

The bushes rustled again, and again they all looked around. Toot, who had been at the edge of the capture scene from the beginning, silently slipped into the blackness, unnoticed.

"What was that?" Dean murmured, peering in the direction of the noise.

"I'll check it out," Godfrey said, slowly rising. "Maybe it's just the wind."

"Miller, we're losing time," Tannenbaum pleaded. "I've been tracking these people for a year. You're just getting in the way. Let me go!"

"First, let's look in your little bag of tricks," Dean said, reaching for the fallen sack. "Frenchie, give a shout if our good friend tries anything …"

He froze with horror. Godfrey and Frenchie looked up and their mouths dropped open. Tannenbaum sat up, rubbing his lip, looking around with puzzlement. Then he too, stiffened with fear.

Killer and the Death Masters stood menacingly before them. They were dressed in black and were holding long knives. Handguns glinted out from under their belts. In the moonlight their faces appeared vague and ghostly.

One of them looked long and hard at Dean, and then tapped his leader. Dean squinted quizzically at the man, then cringed when he recognized him.

"That's him, Killer," Diablo said, pointing. "The one in the apartment."

Both groups seemed equally unprepared for this encounter, and a thick silence surrounded them as they exchanged stares. Godfrey was the first to recover. He walked in front of Dean and faced the intruders.

In the near darkness Killer didn't at first recognize his old partner. When he finally did, he was visibly shocked. So were his companions. This was something they had not even remotely considered.

"Good evening, gentlemen," Godfrey said calmly.

"Godfrey, Godfrey, is that you?" Killer asked incredulously.

"Long time, no see, amigo."

"What are you doing here?" the gang leader asked again, not even trying to hide his confusion.

Godfrey paused. Only Dean seemed to sense that his mind was racing for an answer.

"Helping out a buddy, that's all. Not causing any trouble ..."

"You're helping him out?" Killer asked, starting to recover. He looked at Dean contemptuously. "Godfrey, you sure have changed ..."

"Dean's cool, man."

"Well, your cool buddy Dean, he just killed two of my men. Gouged out their eyes, slit their throats. We don't like that, Dean."

"Self defense, that's all," Godfrey said patiently.

"And I hear he's the one who's been hunting us down."

"That's your man over there," Godfrey said, gesturing at

Tannenbaum. "He goes by the name of Doctor X. Just let us go, we won't cause any problems."

"Him? Doctor X?" Killer asked, nodding towards Tannenbaum, who had struggled to his feet. "The one who's been using us for guinea pigs?"

"That's right," Godfrey answered. Tannenbaum remained silent.

Killer looked back at his companions, and then at his captives.

"Man, this is like Christmas and Saturday night rolled into one," he said with a cold grin. "It's gonna be fun killing both of you …"

"Don't you dare," Frenchie said defiantly, moving out of the shadows. She took a hold of Dean's arm.

Killer couldn't believe his eyes.

"Frenchie? Damn, what is going on tonight?"

"Don't you mess with us."

"My old Frenchie," Killer said softly. "I used to date her. Man, it's been a long time."

Instantly, he snapped out of his reverie.

"Why are you here?" he demanded. "What the fuck are you and Godfrey doing with these people?"

"We don't have to tell you," she snapped, clutching Dean's arm more tightly.

"Don't give me your mouth," Killer snarled. "Old times don't mean shit to me."

"Look, we're on the same side, whether you believe me or not," Godfrey explained, his voice steady. "We chasing the same people you are. This old guy seems to be their leader. Frenchie was just along for the ride."

Killer looked at Godfrey mockingly.

"Ahh, thanks for being on my side, but I really don't think we need your help."

He walked to Dean, ignoring Frenchie at his side.

"So you killed Snake and Ghost," he said. "How could a *nothing* like you do it? I'm gonna save you for last."

He turned and walked up to Tannenbaum. The two men were of equal height and stared at each other eye to eye.

"And you, Doctor X, you're gonna tell me what you did to my men, and why, and then I'm gonna conduct some experiments on you. How about that?"

"Sir, I've done nothing to you or your men, and I'm *not* the one you seek," Tannenbaum said. "Allow me to make a proposition."

Dean was secretly impressed at Tannenbaum's coolness. He does know how to handle himself, he thought.

"Make it fast."

"I'll make it very fast. Let me go, do what you want with them, and I'll give you my bank card and all my cash. We're talking about a lot of money."

Dean looked around, and noticed that Toot was gone.

"Let you 'go?'" Killer asked. "Where are *you* going?"

"To a cabin down this path. There's some very important equipment I've got to get my hands on. And I just may run into Doctor X. Hopefully, all this commotion hasn't blown my cover. So, my good man, do we have a deal?"

Killer glanced at his men, who were standing around awkwardly. They didn't seem quite as fearsome here in the forest, being completely out of their element. They had all gotten lost wandering in the brush, and it had sapped their confidence. Killer realized this was not the time to hire himself out to the enemy.

He violently kneed Tannenbaum in the groin. The man doubled over as if shot, and as his head was moving downward, Killer instantly landed an uppercut to his face. Tannenbaum crashed to the ground, writhing in agony. Killer leaned over and pulled him up by his shirt back to a standing position. The older man grimaced with pain.

"Here's my counter-proposal," Killer snarled. "We're all go to the cabin. You are gonna take us. And you'll give us all your money and whatever 'equipment' is up there. And then you're gonna die! So, my good man, do *we* have a deal?"

He spat loudly in Tannenbaum's face and pushed him several feet back. Tannenbaum reeled backwards but kept on his feet. He leaned against a tree, nearly sobbing with pain.

Killer then turned to Godfrey.

"You take Frenchie and get out of here. We're taking over."

"Killer, let this one go," Godfrey said, indicating Dean with his hand. "Do it for me."

Killer signaled his men, who had been watching intently. "Grab the old man and the punk doctor," he said. "We're going for a walk."

The gang leader turned to Godfrey. The men, each huge and thickly muscled, seemed to tower over the others as they faced each other.

"I am doing something for you," Killer said. "I'm letting you and Frenchie go. That's my gift. This closes my account with you, Godfrey. I don't owe you nothing no more. As for the little doctor here, he's all mine. In fact, this might be as good a time as any to kill him. Yeah, I'll put on a benefit performance. Turn around, Frenchie, unless you're in the mood to see a lot of red."

"To get him you're going to have to go through me," Godfrey said quietly.

In the silvery darkness his words were almost visible with their electricity. The Death Masters were stunned. Godfrey, the legend of the streets, had gone over to the other side.

"What are you saying?" Killer asked, his voice high-pitched with shock. "Man, you would defend one of them?"

"A friend is a friend."

"Godfrey, this is your last chance to side with your brothers."

"I am with my brothers," Godfrey replied softly.

Killer looked at his old comrade. They had grown up together, served in the military together, and had thereafter shortly formed their gang. Soon, the Death Masters ruled the streets, and they all had become rich and notorious, living lavishly and to the last penny. Throughout the years they had remained close, more like brothers than friends.

Killer remembered how hurt he was when Godfrey left the gang. "It's wrong and I just can't do it anymore," Godfrey had said. No reasoning or begging would budge him. When he departed, unarmed and penniless, Killer privately sent word around: Don't ever mess with Godfrey, King of the Death Masters. That was his unspoken, secret present. He felt then as he felt now, heartache that Godfrey, the only person he had ever loved, had left him.

Rage now started to boil within Killer, as he realized the dimensions of this betrayal. Even in the darkness, the change was visible, and the Death Masters looked on, mesmerized.

Killer took one step closer to Godfrey, who calmly stood his ground. Their chests nearly touched. They locked eyes, each poised for combat.

Suddenly, Tannenbaum grabbed his sack and bolted past his captors, who were totally engrossed by the confrontation taking place. He raced down the path toward the cabin, and in seconds had melted into the darkness.

Stunned by his boldness, everyone watched him disappear. Then, with a roar of anger, Killer charged after him, Diablo one step behind.

The remaining Death Masters, sixteen in number, looked bewildered. They stood there uneasily, not knowing what to do with Dean, and especially Godfrey, who was larger than life to them, thanks largely to Killer's penchant for glorifying talks about the "good old days," which usually co-starred this man before them.

"What should we do?" one of them asked. He pointed with his knife in Dean's direction.

"We go to the cabin, like Killer said," another said nervously. "No sense waiting here. You guys, lead the way. And no messing around."

They pulled Dean and Frenchie to the front of the party, and respectfully touched Godfrey's arm, indicating that he join them. Godfrey shrugged and joined his two friends.

"Lead the way," the man with the knife said. "We're watching your backs."

The group began to trudge up the trail, flashlights off, no one having any significant idea of what lay ahead.

Dean held on to Frenchie. He moved quickly, being fairly adept at night walks, having been on several. Godfrey, with his catlike grace, easily kept up. Not so the gang members behind them, who were completely inept in this terrain. The ultimate urban creation, here they seemed almost comical. None had ever been on so much as a daytime hike, and almost immediately they began to fare badly, stumbling on rocks and scratching their faces on overhanging branches. Ironically, most of them, who lived and fought by night, were afraid of the dark. Soon they were left behind, panting and cursing with false bravado, completely oblivious to their former captives.

Within minutes Dean, Frenchie and Godfrey were far ahead, with not so much as a trace of the Death Masters anywhere. When they realized what had happened they began walking even faster. After a while they slowed down. It was apparent to Dean that the gang behind them was by now far away, very likely having veered off onto a side path. Though they seemed to be out of the picture, Killer's threats rang out in his mind and still, somewhere out there, was Doctor X.

Godfrey put his massive hand on Dean's shoulder and signaled for them to stop.

"Listen, I want you two to go back to the car. Otherwise, you're both going to die. Right now, Killer and Diablo are probably cutting up that old man, and they'll do even worse to you. Point me in the right direction. I'll go up the cabin alone, and I'll destroy whatever equipment is there—whatever looks important. I just can't help you against those two guys, they're too much for me."

"Thanks for helping me back there," Dean said. "I really owe you. For everything."

"Don't worry about it. Just go away believing that good people come in all flavors. And remember to tell your kids—you two should have some great ones. Anyway, get ready to cut out. Walk away fast and walk away quiet. Go to that post office at noon every day for the next week. If I make it I'll meet you there."

"I'm not going," Dean said quietly.

"What are you talking about?" Godfrey asked. "There are too many people after you—Killer, Doctor X, all their men. I can't protect you any more."

"Then let me protect you," Dean replied.

"I'm coming along, too," Frenchie said.

Godfrey looked at both of them and nodded.

"Okay, then. Anyway, it is a nice night for a walk."

chapter 60

The trio inched their way along the path, lights off. Aside from an occasional rustle in the bushes, which would instantly freeze them in their tracks, all was still.

Things had been happening so rapidly that Dean had stopped trying to analyze them—he was just riding the flow of events, wherever they led. It reminded him of the roller coaster ride—it was pointless fighting the turns and curves and plunges, so after a while he forced himself to enjoy them.

"How's it going, Frenchie?" he asked quietly. Godfrey had gone a few feet in front of them. They were alone.

"All right, I guess," she answered. There was a trace of weariness in her voice, which he decided to ignore.

"You're doing great."

"I wish I was tougher and could help you, Dean."

"You're plenty tough."

"No, I'm able to absorb a lot of suffering, maybe, but that's not tough. Listen to me. When things get too hard, I just turn everything off. I live on dreams and fantasies, it's how I survive. I'll make believe I'm in some castle, all taken care of. I don't even have to be a princess. Just a lady in waiting, that'd be good enough. And every day I go through the motions of a life, scratching out the dreariest existence possible. You want to know something? When we were trapped in that basement you wished the whole thing was a dream. For me, being there with you was my dream come true. Not very mature, is it? Dean, I wish I had so much more to offer you."

She started crying, the moonlight making her tears run silvery paths down her face. Dean stopped walking and hugged her. She threw her arms around him and held him tightly.

"Don't leave me, Dean," she whispered.

"We'll find a castle some day, Frenchie," Dean said.

"I'm sorry I knew Killer. I'm sorry for all that."

"You were what you were. And now you are what you are. Things, and people, change. I did."

He kissed her. Frenchie's face was cool and wet, and when it touched Dean's face still swollen and puffy from his beating, it almost made him jump.

"Come on, we're almost there," he whispered.

Hand in hand, they walked along the forest path, carefully stepping over the underbrush that seemed much thicker around here.

"It shouldn't be too long now," Dean said. "We're almost …"

He stopped when he saw Godfrey standing very still a few feet up the path. Something was wrong. "What's going on?" Dean said with rising alarm, approaching his friend.

Then he saw the guns.

Diablo stood before them, pointing a gun inches from Godfrey's head. Killer leaned against a tree, smiling at them. Dean could only see Godfrey's back, but he could sense his tension.

"Thanks for joining us," Killer said.

He walked over to Dean, put a thickly muscled arm around him and guided him until the doctor was standing alongside Godfrey.

"Hello again, buddy," Killer said, poking Dean in the ribs. "The old man got away, but you'll do just fine. Have you decided how you want to die? I'm open to suggestions."

"You leave him alone," Frenchie snapped, moving forward.

"Shut your mouth," Killer snarled, backhanding her as she approached, knocking her down.

Dean rushed at Killer in a rage, but Godfrey moved faster and restrained him. Diablo kept his gun trained on the two of them.

"Easy, man," Godfrey whispered, nudging Dean back a few feet. "He'll kill you. Wait for better odds."

"Godfrey, don't ruin my night," Killer said cheerfully. "This man wants to defend his lady's honor, to …"

The gang leader stopped, listening to his words.

"You were about to defend her," he said to Dean. "You two have something going? You two?"

He turned to Frenchie, who was slowly getting off the ground.

"Him? This piece of shit? This faggot doctor?"

"He's a good man," she said defiantly. "I'm his woman."

"You're his cleaning girl is what you are! He wouldn't know what to do with a woman. I'm gonna show him right now. I'm gonna beat him in front of you, and then I'm gonna take you right here. It'll be like old days, remember? You used to moan for my bone, scream for my cream …"

"Shut up!" she shrieked.

"You shut up!" he yelled, smacking her again, knocking her back.

"You pig!" Dean shouted. "You filthy pig!"

With all his might he broke free from Godfrey's hold and stepped in front of Frenchie. He glared at Killer, fists clenched. The gang leader looked down at him with a maniacal gleam. His huge muscles twitched. And then he chuckled coldly.

"It's like a buffet dinner," he said. "I don't know where to begin. Before you die, answer me, what is she to you."

"I love her," Dean said slowly.

"Frenchie?" Killer said.

Blood was dripping from her mouth to her shirt. Frenchie ignored it.

"Dean, I love you," she cried out. "I love you so much."

Killer looked from Dean to Frenchie and then back. For a moment Dean imagined there was a haunted, sad look in his eyes, but then it passed, replaced by an evil glow. Then, with lightning speed, he grabbed Dean by the throat with one hand, his arm outstretched. His grip tightened, and he began to strangle the terrified doctor.

Dean made desperate punching motions, not even coming close, and then he clutched the giant hand around his neck, vainly trying to pry it loose. Killer purposely let just enough air get through his hold, just enough to keep his victim alert. Harsh choking sounds filled the nighttime air.

Just as Dean felt waves of blackness begin to wash over him, Killer let go. Dean crumpled to the ground, retching and coughing. Frenchie, who had been watching in horror, ran over and put her arms around him. Killer moved closer, towering over them.

"Move off him, bitch. I'm just getting warm."

"Lay off him, Killer."

Godfrey's words cut through the air. Everyone turned to look at him, except Dean, who remained on the ground, gasping for air.

"What did you say?" Killer asked.

"I think it's time I reminded you who was the boss. Back off."

In utter amazement, Killer and Diablo watched Godfrey walk over. The big man lifted Dean up as easily as if he were a rag doll and propped him against a tree. Frenchie followed behind them.

Godfrey looked deeply into Dean's eyes. Dean's mind snapped back into focus. Something about Godfrey's demeanor seemed very strange.

"You two run when we start to fight," Godfrey whispered. "Don't argue. Go in different directions, each of you. And don't look back."

Dean and Frenchie looked at each other, each saying with their eyes, I'll meet you at the cabin.

Godfrey turned to the Death Masters. Killer's face was a mixture of bewilderment and outrage. Diablo shifted uneasily, totally at a loss. He had joined the gang when Godfrey was at the height of his power. And Godfrey had never known it, but his walking away had only added to his mystique.

"He belongs to me," Killer warned. "Get out of the way. And then get ready, ex-brother, because you're next."

Killer moved toward Dean, who backed up against the tree. As he neared, Godfrey sidestepped and blocked his way. The two men bumped chests and stood their ground, inches apart, fully mobilized. To Dean it seemed as if two titans were beginning to war.

"Last chance, man, last chance," Killer hissed.

Godfrey took a deep breath and pushed the other man back three feet.

Enraged at having lost face, Killer snapped into an attack position. Godfrey assumed a defensive stance. They slowly began to circle.

Suddenly, with near blinding speed, Killer shot forward, and the two men seemed to explode together.

"Run!" Godfrey screamed.

Dean and Frenchie shot out of the clearing, running at full speed. Immediately they were swallowed by the dark, forbidding forest, each going in a different direction, neither looking back.

chapter 61

Killer and Godfrey crashed heavily onto the ground, punching and clawing. Godfrey remembered from the old days that Killer was at best up close; his inner wrist was already bleeding from his opponent's sharpened thumbnail. He knew that he had to get up. He chopped Killer in the throat and scrambled to his feet.

The two men circled warily, ignoring blood trickling from newly inflicted wounds. Suddenly Killer charged, and as Godfrey moved to dodge, Killer reversed his feint, moved to the side, and smashed two punches into Godfrey's face. Godfrey staggered, but quickly countered with a vicious kick to Killer's stomach, knocking the wind out of him. Then they exchanged several punches, all landing with devastating accuracy.

The two suddenly resumed their death dance, all the while snorting and spitting out the blood that was running freely down their faces. They each realized that only one of them would emerge from this fight alive. Diablo looked on numbly, hypnotized by the battle.

"Moses, give it up," Godfrey taunted, using Killer's old name. "You're a loser, and you're gonna burn in hell."

"You're the dead man Godfrey."

"I saw your mama on her last day," Godfrey said, panting heavily. "She died crying. She died with a broken heart because of you."

"Shut up!" Killer screamed.

"And you're never gonna see her, because you're gonna burn."

"Shut up!"

"Make me," Godfrey taunted.

With a roar Killer charged Godfrey, who kicked him in the face. Killer stiffened in pain and then received a brutal kick to his chest. He quickly recovered and responded with a ferocious combination of jabs and hooks, knocking Godfrey back. Godfrey hit back, and the two then stood toe to toe, trading volley after volley of blows.

Within seconds both were drenched in blood, their own and that of the other. Their faces were barely recognizable, especially Godfrey's, due to Killer's studded rings, sharpened in order to tear flesh. Breathing was excruciating due to the body blows, and each winced with every motion. Still, they battled on. Diablo stared numbly at the two street gods locked in mortal combat, awed by the fury of their violence, by the thundering power of their attacks.

Suddenly, Godfrey jumped back, frantically rubbing his eyes, blinded by a torrent of blood running down his forehead. In that moment Killer pounced upon the opening, smashing Godfrey in the temple with his last remaining strength. Godfrey fell to his knees. Killer's knee crashed into his face. Godfrey rolled backwards and lay still.

Killer staggered over. Blood from several gashes poured freely down his face and dripped on his former comrade. He was in agony from his chest injuries and was unable to catch his breath. He had also lost vision in one eye, one of Godfrey's punches having slammed directly into it. With supreme effort he struggled to stand erect and appear forceful, but he tottered with pain and weakness. Diablo rushed over to hold him steady.

"I warned him," Killer hissed through broken teeth. "He wouldn't shut up."

"Come on and sit down, you're hurt bad," Diablo pleaded, leading his wounded leader to a nearby fallen tree.

They had gone a few feet, when they heard Godfrey's voice behind them.

"Killer, you didn't make me shut up."

Killer whirled around, grimacing in pain. To his horror, he saw that Godfrey had risen to his knee, and was looking at him through eyes nearly swollen shut.

Killer shrugged off Diablo's guiding hand and he shuffled back to his enemy, panting heavily. With all his might he punched Godfrey in the side of the head, who grunted and fell over. Killer tried to bend over and finish him off, but the pain in his chest was too severe, and he was too proud to ask his lieutenant for help. Grimacing in pain, he straightened up.

"Let's get out of here," he wheezed. He was having trouble catching his breath.

As he stiffly started to walk down the path, half blind and desperately short of breath, he heard Godfrey's voice again. It sounded as if it was coming from a grave.

"I'm still talking."

Killer went wild with anger. He turned around and saw Godfrey lying on the ground, his head turned towards him, his eyes staring hatefully.

He staggered back to his fallen opponent, no longer able to will away the pain. He felt too weak to strike out anymore.

"Diablo, give me your knife," he rasped.

"Let me do it for you, Killer," Diablo pleaded.

"Give me your knife," the gang leader commanded.

In a second a long knife was in his hand. Its razor-sharp blade glistened dully in the moonlight.

The gang leader sank heavily to his knees and moved the knife over Godfrey's face. Godfrey looked at the blade, and then at Killer, and smiled. He seemed to be at peace with himself.

"I'm going to cut your eyes out first, and then your tongue," Killer said. "And then we'll see who shuts up."

He aimed at Godfrey's left eye. He held the blade directly over the lower lid, and then began to slowly plunge it in.

The point entered the skin without resistance, and a small trickle of blood burst from the opening. The hand trembled slightly, and a small gash now appeared, allowing more blood to flow out. And then the knife pulled away and fell to the ground, clanging slightly against a pebble when it landed.

Killer died instantly, the long arrow crashing through his skull as if it were a piece of fruit. He hit the ground with a thud and lay there motionless. Diablo looked around him, in a state of total confusion. A moment later, two arrows struck him simultaneously in the chest, penetrating deeply. He collapsed in pain and panic, thrashing wildly. In a few moments he became very still.

Toot and three Indians emerged from the dense underbrush. He ran over to Godfrey, who was losing consciousness, and sat down, cradling him in his arms. The other men walked up and spoke in hushed tones to Toot, who nodded. He got up, and together, they with a slight effort lifted the huge man up and carried him away. The two motionless bodies lay crumpled on the forest path, the cool moonlight painting them a dim silver.

chapter 62

Dean ran through the darkness, his flashlight abandoned during his encounter with Killer. He had veered off the main path, and found himself crashing through light brush, not sure exactly where he was. The moon was his only bearing, and it gave him a rough idea of his general direction, but little else. More than once his shoe would catch on a vine, and he would stagger and fall. Soon he was drenched with sweat, his face and arms scratched and his ragged outfit ever more torn from branches that came at him from all sides.

After a while he re-emerged on a small trail. It seemed to go toward the campsite, he thought. He started moving cautiously along it, semi-crouched, looking about in all directions, painfully aware how treacherous the woods could be.

Dean wondered what had happened to Godfrey and fought the urge to look for him. The guy wouldn't have left me, he thought. Even with their guns.

Pausing, he turned and studied the dense underbrush from where he had come. I could never hope to find him, he sadly thought. Or Frenchie, for that matter. It's up to me now.

He decided to head for the campsite. Keep your eye on the big picture, he forced himself to think.

When he heard the shots crackling directly in front of him he dropped to the ground. As unversed as he was in these matters, he could sense that they weren't aimed at him. He thought of Frenchie and rose, charging down the path, unmindful of the noise he was making. If they can shoot their guns, he reasoned anxiously, I can crack a few twigs.

He ran as fast as he could, and when he hit the small clearing he froze in mid-stride, nearly falling over from his momentum. Crawling behind a bush, he peeked out to view the scene before him.

Two Death Masters lay on the ground. The rest milled around nervously, guns in each hand, looking around in fear. Dean could make out shadowy figures all around. A Death Master stepped forward and aimed his gun at one. Before he could fire, an arrow whistled through the air and shot into his neck. With a gasp he fell backward, twitching violently.

Although it was nighttime, the moonlight etched the fear on their faces. They're too scared to fight, Dean thought, and too scared to escape. They're sitting ducks where they are.

"Back off, you fuckers, or you're dead meat," one of them screamed, brandishing a pistol. "I'm gonna start counting."

Dean heard his voice quavering and knew, as he was sure the shadows did, that the man was terrified.

One of the shadows stepped forward and hurled a spear deep into the gunman's chest. He grabbed at it wildly, staggered forward, and crashed to the ground, pushing the tip through his back. After attempting to get up he collapsed face down, breathing heavily. The night made the blood pooling around him look black.

The remaining Death Masters huddled together and conferred. The shadowy forms all around were silent and motionless. The creamy moonlight bathed the entire scene with ghostlike whiteness.

Then the Death Masters started their attack, all of their guns blazing at once. Bullets whistled and ricocheted everywhere; one grazed Dean's face as he hit the ground. The entire area seemed to erupt into explosions, the noise overwhelming. Dean looked up and saw the clearing filled with smoke and flashes of light.

The Death Masters fired away almost continuously, in every direction, pausing only to reload. There was no way of telling how much damage they were doing, but for a few moments they ruled the woods.

Grunts and screams emanated from the darkened perimeters. The gun-men seemed to grow stronger with the noise, the power of the streets overcoming that of the forest.

But soon a hail of arrows and spears answered in a volley of their own, with deadly accuracy. Four of the shooters fell instantly, and a fifth dropped to his knees, and arrow in his groin. He screamed in pain and anger, firing wildly all around him. A spear quickly found his neck, killing him as he knelt.

The other Death Masters kept firing, desperately aiming at any-thing moving. Several were hit with arrows, but they fought on. Then, one by one, they ran out of ammunition, and their guns started click-ing. An eerie silence ensued, all the more striking after the bedlam of the last minute. Dean watched in fascination as the last of the Death Mas-ters dropped their firearms and pulled out long knives. Coolly, they walked forward, directly toward the group of shadows that was coalesc-ing in front of them.

Screaming their war cry, the gang plunged into battle, flailing all around them furiously. There was a hideous outpouring of shouts and snarls and screams, and in the grayness Dean could make out the shape-less forms locked in hand to hand combat, all fighting to the death.

A minute later, all was still. The Death Masters lay on the ground, motionless. The shadows stood all around them.

This is your chance, Dean thought. While they lick their wounds, get to the cabins.

Backing his way out of the area, he crawled until he reached an-other small trail. With nothing to lose, he rose and began charging down it. Perhaps because his night vision had fully adapted to the darkness, or because he was driven by love or fear or desperation, his feet barely seemed to touch the ground, as he ran with astounding grace. In min-utes he had reached the path's end. He stopped, breathing heavily, and surveyed the scene.

The cabins were in the clearing. The site appeared deserted, but signs of recent habitation were everywhere, with large cartons piled by several doors. Everyone went off to fight the gang, he reckoned. It's now or never.

He ran out of the woods and into the clearing, hoping there were no guards. He approached the cabins, which stood in a row. The first three seemed empty, though it was difficult to see inside. The fourth had its windows blackened. He tried to peer inside to no avail. Suddenly there were shouts from the nearby trees. The guards were returning. Keep going, he said to himself, there's no turning back now.

He ran to the door and grabbed the handle, both surprised and grateful that it was unlocked. Looking back, he could make out shadows in the distance. He took a deep breath, grit his teeth and entered.

chapter 63

Dean rushed into the cabin, fists clenched, ready to fight. Instead, he found himself in a quiet, smoky room that glowed a faint orange from several torches on the walls. Two chairs and a small table were in the very center, and a mattress lay by the corner. A pot bellied iron stove gently radiated heat. On top of it sat a small, steaming ceramic pot, covered by a brightly colored cloth.

He locked the door, hoping it would give him extra time and walked over to the stove. After having been outside for so long, with its over-whelming grayness, the gentle hues of the room, with its quiet and warmth, had a deeply soothing effect on him, and he resisted the im-pulse to sit down and rest. He suddenly felt very, very tired.

He lifted a corner of the cloth covering the pot. There was a famil-iar aroma, but Dean couldn't place it. He wondered, was this it? Could this be the substance he had been seeking—the potion of Doctor X?

The thought made him smile. He started to giggle, and then laugh. The more he looked into the pot, the more he laughed. Soon he was unable to control himself. So it's come down to this, tears running down his face. All the death and pain, all the craziness, all for a vat of chicken soup. I don't know whether to destroy it or help myself to a bowl. Give me some crackers and I'll take over the world.

He collapsed in a heap, laughing and crying, not caring if anyone outside heard him. Suddenly, a figure on the mattress stirred, moving slightly. Dean snapped back to attention, looking around wildly. His hysteria evaporated as quickly as it had appeared. The figure groaned, adjusted the dark woolen blanket over it and lay still again. Dean rubbed the tears away with a dirt smeared forearm and stared at it. For a moment he felt anger at having his privacy invaded, then he pushed the feeling away, knowing it was illogical. He started to crawl over. The war goes on, he thought.

On all fours, silently, he inched his way forward. Don't kill, he thought, get information. And don't be nice, there's no time. Careful, careful ...

He ripped off the blanket and prepared to strike. Then he stared, mouth open in disbelief.

"Connigan!"

The scientist bolted upright, his eyes wild and his lips retracted into a snarl, revealing his teeth. Dean jumped to his feet, fearful, but instantly recovered. It's too late to be afraid, he said to himself, thinking of Godfrey. Things have gone too far.

"What are you doing here?" Dean snapped.

"Loving everything, always vibrating energy, mustering enthusiasm," Connigan hissed. "A lucid oracle never exists."

Dean's mind raced, as he repeated the words over in his mind. Connigan was talking in code.

"Screw you and your poetry," he snapped, poking the large man in the chest. "Talk to me. What are you doing?"

A thin line of saliva trickled from the corner of Connigan's mouth. He looked straight ahead.

"Slithering asps, vipers, in nighttime gambits, throwing hellacious elixirs," he hissed. "Writhing over rocks, loveless, demonic,"

He closed his eyes, and began rocking back and forth. Dean looked on in frustration. Suddenly, rage hit him. This man has no right to kill me or anyone, he thought. He has no right ...

Dean went down on one knee. He grabbed Connigan by the shoulders and violently shook him.

"Stop it!" the doctor screamed. "Stop it this minute!"

Connigan paused and turned to Dean. Inexplicably, his eyes had cleared. There was now an air of unspeakable sadness about him. Dean's arms fell to his sides as he studied the man before him. He saw ~~before~~ a lost

~~soul~~ ~~the man~~ in deep torment, fighting a valiant but losing struggle against some demon or demons. Without knowing why, he forgave Connigan.

"Why, why did you do it?" Dean asked gently, his eyes filling with tears.

"Because there is pain in the world," Connigan whispered. "Because things didn't work out as they should have."

"And for that you would kill all the babies in their cribs?"

"It's too late for this discussion," Connigan said, turning away.

Dean sat down on the mattress, in front of the scientist.

"It's not too late, and you know it. They're releasing the virus at midnight, aren't they?"

Connigan's face twisted in pain.

"Yes," his lips moved. "I'm sorry."

"Professor, did you leave that book in the ER on purpose?" Dean asked softly. "Did part of you want me to stop you?"

"I'm sorry. I'm sorry, I'm sorry, I'm sorry, I'm sorry …"

"Then tell me how to dismantle the bomb" Dean said more forcefully. He realized he was beginning to lose Connigan.

Connigan closed his eyes for a few seconds, and then opened them. He stared at Dean, not blinking. Dean recoiled, knowing it was too late.

"Come back," he begged. "Connigan, tell me how to stop this horrible thing. Please."

Connigan's eyes bored into him.

"Not tonight, darling," he cackled. "I have a headache."

Just then the door seemed to bend inward with an unseen force. Dean sprang to his feet and raced over to the pot, kicking it over. At that moment the groaning wood exploded and men rushed in. Dean charged into them, trying to blast his way through and make it to the door. They grabbed him and wrestled him to the ground. He thrashed violently, trying to punch and kick them. Go on, kill me, you bastards, his mind screamed. He felt their punches and clubs raining down on him, but curiously felt little pain, rather only a deepening weakness and remoteness from the entire scene. His last sensation before losing consciousness was that of floating over them, looking down on the beating, imagining himself an actor in a wordless play. He saw himself being rolled over and tied up. And then everything went black.

chapter 64

Cold water splashed into Dean's face, shocking him into wakefulness. He choked as it went into his nose and down his mouth, and he sat upright trying to catch his breath.

The discomfort was replaced by a moment of panic; in the darkness he had totally lost his bearings, he no longer knew where he was, or what he was doing here. Then, suddenly, everything that had happened came back abruptly into focus.

"Get up," a voice commanded.

Dean looked up at the nearly invisible silhouette of a man in front of him. They were outdoors now, but the moon was hidden by the trees, and the night's darkness was that much deeper. He shut his eyes tight, then opened them widely, trying to let as much light in as possible. He sensed he had been moved some distance, and noted that the ground was gently sloping. He figured that they were at the base of a small mountain, one of the first of a large chain, one that extended for many miles, deep into the vast forests further north.

"Get up," his captor repeated, more harshly. This time, without waiting for Dean to comply, arms roughly hauled him to his feet. It took him a few seconds to regain his balance.

"Start walking," a man behind him ordered.

The small party, with Dean in the middle, wended its way through a maze of moonlit boulders. Though he spent most of his efforts struggling to walk in near darkness, Dean thought he counted ten men. They were silent, and their faces weren't visible, but he imagined them to be the same people who had captured him in the abandoned building several days before. Somehow both attacks on him had the same feel, a curious holding back on their part, almost as if the violence had been tinged with a palpable gentility.

There was no trace of any path, and Dean had no idea of how far they had carried him. Although completely in the open, they were totally alone, especially at night, amid the vast emptiness of the giant park. Even at summer's peak they probably would have been unnoticed, as they were far from any normal trail. In addition, the giant boulders all around them now shielded them from view.

Without warning they stooped at a small crack in the side of a seemingly solid rocky wall. Two men got on their hands and knees and crawled through, instantly disappearing. The other motioned for Dean to follow. He halted, looking into the opening with disbelief. A cave, he thought. Connigan said something about one—I should have guessed. A hard jab in his back forced the issue, and he lowered himself to the ground. They can kill me whenever they want, he thought wearily as he crawled inside the hole. There's no point in resisting now.

Almost immediately he found himself in an underground passageway. With no idea where he was going, relying only on the sounds of the men in the front of him, he kept moving forward. The silvery darkness of the outside quickly evaporated, and they soon were in complete blackness.

The crawlway veered sharply upward and to the left, and simultaneously became larger. The small party halted while several men lit torches, and then they proceeded, at first in a crouch and then, finally, fully erect.

The crystalline walls of the tunnel sparkled in the light. Dean saw no distinguishing marks, or signs of use, and surmised that few if any people even knew of its existence. The path twisted and turned, at several points forking, the little group unhesitatingly selecting a route. It was obvious that they were well aware of where they were going; Dean knew only that they were deep in the mountain by now. He was hopelessly lost ████, and knew it would be nearly impossible for anyone to now find them. For better or worse, my lot is cast with these people, he thought. And something tells me the time has come to meet Doctor X.

chapter 65

It was impossible to gauge time or distance. Eventually they entered a large, theater-shaped chamber, lit by several torches. In front of one wall, which gave Dean the impression of a stage, was a bubbling stream. It was fed by a thick seam of shimmering water that emerged from a crack high up in the wall, which cascaded down as if a miniature waterfall. The collected water ran along the wall's length and disappeared into the stony floor. Aside from a small entrance at the other end, the area was perfectly enclosed. Shadowy figures aimed bows and arrows at them from behind several large boulders around them.

Dean blinked in surprise when he saw that alongside the stream was a giant version of the ceramic pot he had seen in the cabin. It rested on carefully placed logs, which burned gently. With its shape and gray and red earth tones, it appeared perfectly natural in this setting. Two warriors, dressed in loincloths, their faces painted, stood by its side, bows and arrows in their hands. They eyed him coldly as he passed. Dean looked back in astonishment.

"Hi, my darling," Frenchie said.

He whirled around, stunned at the sound. Having traveled in silence through this alien landscape, her voice was as jolting as it was reassuring. She was seated on the floor, cradling Godfrey in her arms. He was nearly unrecognizable from facial injuries, and he lay silently.

"Good to see you, Dean," Godfrey mumbled.

"Oh, God," Dean gasped, breaking ranks with his captors to kneel by them. He lightly touched Frenchie's face.

"I didn't know what happened to you," he said.

"I was running and they just grabbed me," she whispered. "It all happened so fast."

"And look at him," Dean said, with his pain in his voice. "Godfrey, look at you. This is my fault. I should have been there to help you."

"Nah, you did the right thing," Godfrey said. "This was between me and him."

Instinctively, Dean rapidly examined his friend, who appeared to have dozed off. The warriors stared curiously, but left them alone. Their bows remained taut, and aimed at them.

"I guess he's okay," Dean murmured. "He'll need some X-rays if we ever get out of this."

He looked at Frenchie. It was very good to see her.

"Still love me after all this?" he asked quietly.

She leaned over and kissed him. Then she pulled back and smiled at him.

"As far as I can tell, this is one of your average days."

They both laughed.

"I'm so sorry I dragged you into all this," he said.

"That was supposed to be my line," she said.

"I don't think we'll die, Frenchie. They would have killed us by now. There's a reason for all of this."

"That's right, Miller. It's to witness the end of the world."

Dean looked up and saw Tannenbaum a few feet away. His hands were tied in front of him.

"What are you doing here?" Dean asked. "I thought you ..."

At that moment another group of warriors entered from the opposite door, escorting three people into the chamber. They led the trio to where Dean and his party were, and backed away carefully. Dean squinted in disbelief.

"It's impossible," he whispered.

"Doctor Miller, I presume," Finkel said with mock gravity. "And may I present the other members of our lost expedition."

He made a sweeping motion with his head, as if making a grand presentation. Dean's mouth dropped, as Carol sheepishly smiled at him. Ehler averted his eyes, an air of melancholy around him.

"You're in on this?" Dean asked incredulously. "I don't believe this."

Finkel turned to Carol.

"Are we 'in on it?' He's on to us, darling. It's time to activate …"

"Fink, button it," Carol said. "Dean, they caught us days ago."

"Dean, are these your hospital friends?" Frenchie asked in confusion.

"We were hospital friends," Finkel said, "Now we're prison friends. My name's Bob. And this is my prison bride, Carol. We're on our honeymoon. The man sulking over here is Dan Ehler."

"I'm Frenchie."

"Just so you know, we're a unit, the two of us," Dean said, touching her hand. The others eyed her curiously.

"She's too good for you, Dean," Carol finally said.

"You silly children," Tannenbaum growled. "While you're making prom arrangements, they're going to unleash their attack."

"If you'd been truthful from the beginning maybe things would be different now," Dean snapped angrily. "We wouldn't *be* prisoners now, did you ever think of that? And if you can think of something better to do than make prom arrangements, just let me know. Until then, shut up!"

"Dean, did he come with you?" Finkel asked.

"No, we sort of bumped into him in the forest," Dean said. "I thought he was Doctor X. I guess not, huh?"

"Chief, what's going on?" Finkel asked.

"I spent months tracking them down, and you've ruined everything," Tannenbaum replied icily. "Tonight's the night. Those archers are standing next to the poison itself."

"They hauled it out a little while ago," Finkel said, looking at the vat. "I assume they're going to pour it into that stream, which will empty into waters outside this place."

Finkel and Carol sat down. Ehler leaned against a wall, staring at the trickling stream.

"Have long have you been here?" Frenchie asked, keeping her eyes on the water.

"We were grabbed leaving a hotel," Carol answered. "It seems like a million years ago. There aren't any clocks here, you just sort of go by your own biorhythm. And Dan …"

"They took me out of the ER," Ehler said listlessly, sitting down, crossing his legs. "I have no idea why. No one's said anything. I miss my kids so much."

"Did anyone hurt you?" Frenchie asked.

"No, they treat us all right," Ehler said, dejectedly. "They let us walk around the dead end caves unescorted, there's no way to escape. We eat with them, we sleep with them, we basically live with them."

"And we all relieve ourselves in the same place, down at the end of one of these trails," Finkel said. "Dean, have you ever shared a bathroom with thirty-five cavemen?"

"Fink calls it the 'mocha chamber,'" Carol said.

"Darling, I'd call it what they call it, but I don't speak 'Og'"

"Why did they bring you here?" Dean asked.

"I don't know exactly, but I'm sure it has something to do with that stupid book of yours," Finkel said.

"I told you it was on the level."

"Why couldn't you have told someone else?"

"I think we've moved beyond that particular stage by now," Carol said. "Dean, in fifty words or less, what is going on?"

"Yes, Miller, why don't you brief them on your counter-terrorism activities," Tannenbaum sneered.

"You shut up!" Dean snapped.

After recovering from their surprise, they turned back to Dean, more puzzled than ever.

In minutes, he filed them in on the events of recent days. His friends stared warmly at Godfrey and Frenchie. They looked angrily at their chief. He ignored them, staring at the large vat all the while.

"You could have brought the authorities in on this long ago," Ehler said bitterly, glaring at Tannenbaum. "What do you have to say for yourself?"

"Number one, I didn't have the book, so there was nothing concrete to tell them," Tannenbaum snapped. "I just had bits and pieces of information to go on. And number two, go to hell."

"Why can't you be friendly," Frenchie said in exasperation. "It looks like we're on the same side. Obviously you are not Doctor X. Can we work together on this?"

"You clearly are more astute than your colleagues, however meaningless it is at this point. But if you want to make me very happy, just knock over that potion without letting anything spill into the underground spring. When that mixture is ready they're going to pour it into the water. Then it's just a matter of time before it spreads to your friends and mine."

"So what was in the big sack you were carrying?" Dean asked sullenly.

"If you must know, Miller, it was a massive bomb."

Suddenly everyone turned their eyes to the far door. The trickling water made the only sound, but there was the sense of people approaching. At that moment Jungle Man, Mr. Natural and a third, shorter figure, shrouded in a white cloak, entered. The small figure went over to a far corner and sat down on the rock shaped throne. Jungle Man walked over to confer with the archers by the large vat. Mr. Natural approached the captives.

chapter 66

Mr. Natural slowly walked past in silence, looking at them, hands clasped behind his back. He nodded his head slowly, as if reviewing a line of troops. Then he turned around and faced them.

"Good evening, everyone, and thanks for joining us tonight," he drawled.

He looked at Dean.

"Boy, someone sure beat the crap out of you," Mr. Natural said, studying Dean's face.

"I've had better days," Dean replied warily.

"How's your friend," Mr. Natural asked, peering at Godfrey, who seemed to be semi-conscious.

"He'll be okay. Thanks for asking."

"Why wouldn't I ask? I'm not a bad person. No one here is, actually. Actually, as groups go, we're a great collection of genuinely nice people. We're just on the other side of the same coin. And tonight, we're going to flip the coin."

"Flip it, huh?" Ehler said disdainfully. Unlike Dean, he had never liked the security guard.

"That's right, sir, it's our turn now. I'm sure it's a dumb idea, but you know us burnt out hippies. We've got holes in our brains, we're losers. Right? You used to say that about me all the time, remember? It's true, I was listening."

Ehler was silent. He didn't recall saying that, but knew it was distinctly possible.

"Don't worry, I never minded locker room talk," Mr. Natural continued, his voice turning cold. "Hell, you didn't even know me."

"What's going on tonight?" Dean asked. From the corner of his eye he could see Toot seated on a large, flat rock, his legs crossed, observing everything. Toot was unarmed.

"Just like I said, we're going to flip the coin."

"I'm sorry, but what does that mean," Dean said.

Mr. Natural was dressed in a loose fitting, coarsely woven gray outfit, almost medieval in style. The way he and the warriors looked here in this bare cavern made any sense of time and place irrelevant. Dean was having trouble keeping a firm grasp on where he really was. The power of the modern world did not extend here, and he felt as if they had all been hurled into another time and place, far from their own.

Mr. Natural cleared his throat. "I'm glad you asked that, because it's a good lead into my big introduction. I didn't have much practice at this, but here goes.

"About two years ago, I had this dream. God, Odin and Jupiter had a poker game going, you know, something to just pass the eternal time, it was a cosmic thing. Anyway, God was running low on chips, so He decides to put up the Earth as collateral. And you know what? Jupiter laughs. He goes 'Bull-Shit', Earth ain't worth crap no more. If you want to bet, you put up somethin' worth somethin'. God goes, 'what the ....' and He looks for Himself. He'd been away on some important business, and He had left the place in the hands of mortals who, He figured, could be left alone and unsupervised for at least a little while.

"You know what He saw? He sees that His pride and joy, the place where all living things were supposed to live happily ever after, was now a smoking dump, piled high with garbage, and bulging with hungry, diseased masses. Nearly all the people worshipped money, and the ones who had money spent their lives exploiting all the ones who didn't. And it got worse than that. I mean, they were killing fifty animals just to make one fur coat. They were chopping down entire forests because they wanted the trees to make fancy coffee tables.

"Boy, did He ever get mad. 'Damn it all', He says. 'I turn my back on the place for a measly thousand years and look what happens. Now

I got some big time repair work to do. I need to find Me a contractor.'
And then I woke up."

Mr. Natural looked at them, grinning.

"Gee, and they taught us that God didn't play craps with the universe," Finkel said.

"Shut up. Tonight, His work will be done, and all the wrongs will
be righted," Mr. Natural continued, smiling broadly. "This computer
driven House of Babel will be coming down very shortly. We're gonna
push the delete button right here, from this very room. You have been
chosen by Doctor X to be the official 'End of The Modern World' pea-
nut gallery. Feel free to shout and get into the swing of things. This
chamber is completely soundproof from the outside. Would you believe we didn't hear so much as a pop from that gun battle?

"Just one thing," he continued, his face turning more serious. "It
wasn't my idea to bring you here. As far as I'm concerned, you're just
glorified hostages for us in case we're found out, and, damn, am I ever
ready to sacrifice your asses. I wouldn't lose any sleep if any of you tried
something stupid and got killed. But you won't get hurt if you behave.
Talk all you want, but I promise you that there are ten master archers
watching you at this very moment, and they have orders to waste anyone who so much as blinks the wrong way. You won't know what hit
you—I've seen them shoot butterflies out of the air."

The shrouded figure rose from the seat at the other end of the chamber and walked over to Jungle Man. Dean leaned forward, arching his
neck to look at them. Suddenly, he noticed two archers glaring at him.
He sat back instantly.

Mr. Natural walked over to the large vat and uncovered it. Steam
wafted into the air. He removed a thermometer from a pocket and gently placed it inside. After a moment he removed it and nodded at the
hooded figure, who signaled him to back off. Obediently, the large man
eased his way into the background.

The figure walked in before them, facing the party on the ground.
Dean tried to focus on the face, which was slightly visible, but it was too
dark. Then, in one sudden motion, the shroud fell to the ground. Helen
stood before them.

chapter 67

Dean started violently when he saw her, sucking his breath in.

"Helen, what are you doing here?" he gasped.

She surveyed them and the entire room with a serene majesty. The Indians lowered their eyes when she looked their way. Her eyes rested on him. There was a haunted look on her face. She licked her lips and smiled at him.

"Hello, Dean. I knew we'd meet again,"

"Helen, what is going on?"

"Why don't you take a guess, Dean?"

"You're Doctor X, aren't you?" Frenchie asked.

"Maybe," Helen said. "And you must be Frenchie. I've heard about you."

"Frenchie," Dean blurted out incredulously. "There's got to be ..."

"Let her talk, Dean," Helen said with a hint of amusement.

"I figured it was you. You were supposed to meet Connigan in the clinic that night, but you let Dean switch with you because he got sick. That wasn't too bright. Then you tried to get the book from Dean when he found it. He said you were once a psychiatric nurse. You met the professor on a mental ward, didn't you?"

"Maybe," Helen said again, studying the woman on the ground before her.

"I should have told Dean," Frenchie said. "In the book, Connigan says, 'For you I launch a thousand ships into the night.' That's from Marlowe. The beautiful Helen, whose face launched a thousand ..."

"You're Doctor X," Dean mumbled. "Impossible."

"Dean it's quite possible," Helen finally said. Her eyes seemed to burn in the fire's light.

"That's what you call her," Jungle Man said to them gently. "We call her Cassiana, in honor of a great chief who lived in my grandfather's time—a colonist who joined the Cherente tribe, who became one of them and who went on to lead them. And all of you may join us if you wish—all of you—because you are all good people. Which of you is Dan? You? Know that your wife and children received the protection. We tried not to scare them. They're safe in one of our houses. You will be seeing them soon."

Ehler let out a deep breath and looked down. Then he started crying, his body rocking back and forth.

"So, we have quite a group here tonight," Helen continued, pointedly ignoring Frenchie as she addressed the others. "Dean, it's good to see you. You were one of the great 'what-ifs' for me. Maybe some other lifetime, okay? I still can't get over how you got that book. It was crazy switching with you. What a lapse in judgment. It filled me with self-doubts, it made me wonder if, subconsciously, I was trying to fail. It wouldn't have been for the first time.

"And then you broke the code," she went on. "Quite impressive."

"That was Frenchie, she did it," Dean said.

"Really. Good for you, Frenchie," Helen said distantly. "I've seen you once or twice in the hospital. You shoot drugs, don't you?"

"No, lately you could say I'm getting high on life," Frenchie shot back. Her hand found Dean's and squeezed it.

The two women locked eyes.

"Archers, kill this woman," Helen said casually, looking away.

"No!" Dean screamed. He jumped in front of Frenchie, who held onto him tightly. "Kill me, I got her into this."

The archers hesitated, not having a clear target. Quietly, Jungle Man walked over and whispered into Helen's ear. The woman, who was trembling slightly, nodded in agreement.

"All right, no one here will get hurt," she said. "Sorry about that, Frenchie. It must be all this stress that's getting to me."

"Not to mention all this playing God," Tannenbaum added coldly.

"We'll get to that later," Helen said, regaining her composure. "Let's see who else is here, since we have some time. Here we have Godfrey, a half dead hero, a vanishing breed in the age of antiheroes. What a lonely existence you must have. I'm glad you'll survive, the new age will need greatness."

Dean looked at Godfrey, and then at Toot, who was casually touching a spot on his neck. They had the protection all along, he thought.

"And let's not forget Toot over there," Helen said, following Dean's eyes to the man perched on the rock. He waved to her.

"You're going home, Toot. Hang in there just a few more days."

Helen walked up to Finkel, Carol and Ehler.

"You guys are outrageous. All that talk in the ER about the end of the world! Oh, how I wanted to let you in on this. You may hate me, but I love all of you, and I am so glad you'll all be saved."

"I don't hate you," Finkel said.

"Thanks. But you can if you want. It's okay to control your actions but not your feelings. Of course, Fink, you have no feelings—that's your standard line. But if you had any, and you did hate me, it would be all fine with me. Carol, take good care of him, and watch out for the others, you're the toughest of the bunch. Oh, by the way, Bob. We even set a dose aside for Harry. Isn't that cool, you'll be seeing him for years to come."

"I don't even know what to say," Finkel replied dryly.

"Now, who did I leave out? Oh my goodness, Doctor Tannenbaum. The Big Chief himself. How's it going, boss? Wife and kids okay? Four sons, if I remember correctly. Gee, they must be getting big. You must be so proud."

Tannenbaum twisted against his ropes, his face a mask of pure hatred.

"Monster!" he snarled.

"Gee, once upon a time you called me 'Sweetie.' That was the time I brought my little son in to see you. With a little touch of epiglottitis? Remember?"

Tannenbaum stopped, and stared at her in confusion.

"What are you talking about?" he growled. A hint of recognition suddenly flickered across his face and his eyes betrayed a trace of panic.

"Nothing. Everything. I do wish you had been a touch less cavalier that night—we might not be saying our farewells now."

"Helen, answer me, why are you doing all of this," Ehler implored. "Are you getting revenge on the world?"

"Are lions and tigers really that sacred to you?" Carol added.

"These questions, all these questions," Helen said with mock weariness. "And there are so many answers. Which truths do I give you?"

She looked at the ceiling, as if searching for words. The large room was silent except for the constant, almost peaceful trickling sounds made by the underground stream.

"It's funny how the world turns, isn't it," she began. "Dean, can you imagine how different things would have been had you gone home that night and had not met the professor? You wouldn't have been imprisoned, or beaten, or even here right now. But then you would have died in ten or twenty days and, as far as I can tell, not fallen in love. By the way, none of you were meant to receive the antidote. That was improvised along the way, as you kept intruding into our space. We started taking a liking to you. In other words, you were plain lucky.

"When you get down to it, so very much of everything boils down to luck," Helen continued. "The person who loses control of his car and crashes into someone else could just as easily have crashed into you. There's no reason why. It certainly has nothing to do with who is a better person.

"It was like that with my Tommy," she said. "I brought him to a doctor who was overworked and all strung out. He made a bad clinical decision and, poof, no more Tommy. I later found out the other doctor on that night was fresh, and considered to be far superior. It was the middle of the night, and both were free. They told us to go into one of the exam rooms and wait. And I chose the wrong door."

Tannenbaum looked at her. She calmly stared back.

"Sorry," Dean said uneasily.

"Don't be. Things like that put you at a crossroads. You can spend the rest of your life feeling sorry for yourself, and shrivel up with bitterness. Or you can learn how to shrug, and know that it wasn't personal, it was just dumb luck.

"When I realized the universe did not revolve around me, that I was just a chance particle passing through, that I was the result of a quickie my parents had one night, everything changed. Living is great, but I know I'm going to die, just like every person who's ever lived or who ever will live. The details don't mean a thing.

"But you know what does count a lot? The big picture. This big beautiful planet. As far as anyone can tell it's the only one of its kind. And we were destroying it. *Were* destroying it. Past tense. The destruction stops tonight. I couldn't save my little Tommy but as God is my witness I am going to save this world!

"It upsets me that when I read about the devastation of the oceans and forests, and the extinctions of plants and animals. That bothers me a lot. Nature by definition is immortal. What we're doing goes against the very grain of existence."

Dean and Finkel exchanged glances, recalling their cavalier talks in the ER.

"Helen, you've gone crazy," Ehler said, fear in his voice.

"You have to ask yourself, who gives anyone the right to kill elephants for their tusks, or wolves because it's cool, or to displace entire tribes because some corporation wants to use their land for cocoa," Helen went on, ignoring him. "Who has the right to melt the North Pole and wipe out the polar bears? The answer, obviously, is that people with power give themselves the right."

"You will burn in hell if you do this," Ehler warned. "Helen, there's time to stop this."

"No, Dan, there's not. It's too late for you guys. I defected to the other side a few years ago. To the side of the jungle. And to the ancient peoples who lived there in harmony for thousands of years. I fooled you back in the ER, didn't I? Oh, and when I switched sides, boy, did I bring a few secrets along with me."

From a pocket she withdrew a small vial. In it was a thick, bluish liquid. Several warriors pulled their bowstrings taut with readiness, aiming at Dean and his fellow captives, and one knelt before her, dropping to his hands and knees, so that should it drop, it would not break.

"I'd like to introduce my offspring, about eight trillion trillion of them," she said with a gleam. "I love each and every one of them. They have their mother's eyes, don't you think?"

She fluttered her eyelashes at the group, her eyes bulging with emotion.

"Ebola-influenza combo, I bet that's what it is," Finkel said. "I'd put my money on something like that. It would make the most sense."

"Pretty close," Helen said proudly. "We even programmed our own transcriptase. In a basement, no less."

"What's she talking about?" Carol asked Finkel, who was nodding at the beaker, a grudging admiration in his eyes.

"It's a nickname for a DNA polymerase," Finkel whispered. "It controls protein production. I'll tell you the rest in the jungle one day, over a bowl of lizard soup."

"I heard that, and you know, Bob's right," Helen said, smiling. "In more ways than one. By the way, Dean, that's pretty much what you kicked over in the cabin. Some of the guys are really ticked off at you. Cute, very cute."

She laughed loudly, shaking her head.

"You evil monster," Tannenbaum hissed.

"Now, is that any way to talk to a colleague," Helen said, feigning coyness. In a moment her expression changed to that of pure hatred. She glared at him.

"Helen, what exactly are you going to do?" Dean asked.

"All right, let's get down to business," she said, turning to look at him. "I'm actually glad you're all here, it's like the old days. This is the final act, so let's make the most of it. And when we're done, the audience is free to leave.

"In a few minutes we're going to return the earth to a time when the open lands were endless, when nature was so overwhelming and majestic people actually worshipped it. To a time when there was enough food, no crime, no suicide bombers, no unemployment and no artificial ingredients. To a time of perfect harmony.

"Granted, laptops and video games will be lost forever, and people will actually die when they get very old or very sick. But overall, I think the system should work fairly well, as it did for many, many, thousands of years.

"At this moment, nearly all the forests and jungles, and the life in them, are gone. Most inland and coastal waters are little more than cesspools, and the air grows more cancerous every day.

"Today, today alone, an area half the size of this park vanished from the face of the earth and will never come back. It's unstoppable. Every computer calculation and permutation indicates that in less than a hundred years everything will have been consumed, unless nuclear proliferation or global warming brings about the demise even sooner. Either scenario, the slow rotting of the planet or its thermonuclear demise, guarantees one thing—when the ends does arrive, nothing will be salvageable.

"But then along comes a dedicated doctor who finds a cure for what had been an incurable disease," Helen said, caressing the beaker. "This is the medicine for a very sick planet."

She kissed the vial.

"It's a shame so many thousands of cultures and animal species have already been exterminated over the past two centuries," she added softly. "But, as they say, let's not mourn the past, let's go back to it."

"It should take a few thousand years or so to reverse most of the damage, but who's counting," Mr. Natural added. "The forest and most of the endangered species should all bounce back nicely. As for the rats, roaches and other human parasites, well, they're on their own."

He walked over and checked the liquid's temperature. Everyone in the cavern watched motionlessly.

"Doctor X, the time has come," Mr. Natural said solemnly.

Helen straightened and nodded to the assembled warriors, who moved to pre-arranged places. Those who had not already, loaded their bows. She walked over to the large vat. Jungle Man removed the cloth covering.

"I dedicate this to the rain forests, the northern woods and everything in between," she said, raising the beaker. "May all the evil be undone, and may the Earth once again become the paradise it was."

She started to tilt the beaker. A thin line of blue reached the rim of the glass.

At that moment the device Tannenbaum had planted in the woods exploded.

chapter 68

Enormously powerful, the bomb sent a deep rumble into the cave, its shock waves making the ground and walls tremble all around them. Dust, glowing yellow from the torchfires, swirled through the air.

The warriors froze, suspecting an earthquake, half expecting the cavern to collapse and bury them forever. Helen jumped at the sound, totally thrown off guard. Jungle Man moved towards her, a deep concern in his eyes. Godfrey lifted his head, and through swollen eyes looked at Dean.

"If you want that poison, now's your chance," he said.

Dean bolted up and shot towards Helen. The disoriented warriors didn't even notice him. By the time they looked back towards their leader, seconds later, Dean had wrestled control of the beaker and was standing next to Helen, holding his prize high in the air.

"Oh my God!" Helen gasped.

"It was a nice try, Helen," Dean said. "Maybe some other lifetime, okay?"

He tilted the beaker. Slowly, deliberately, he began to pour the mixture on the ground. The blue drops made little splashing noises on the stone floor.

"No, Dean, please don't," Helen whispered.

She put her hands together as if in prayer.

"Please," she begged. She looked deeply into his eyes. A yellowish haze seemed to envelope her, making her appear haunted, ghostlike.

Dean paused and returned her gaze. Helen, what goes on inside your head, he thought, what do your beautiful eyes actually see. You've shaken my faith in myself, in my ability to perceive reality.

"She's a devil, Miller, don't stop!" Tannenbaum roared. "Don't lose your advantage!"

"Archers, take your aim," Mr. Natural commanded sternly. He stared at the blue liquid already on the ground, and at Dean, hatred in his eyes.

Obediently, grateful to amend for the lapse in control, the men raised their bows and targeted the small group, who cringed and bent towards the ground. The taut sounds of stretching leather filled the room.

"If one more drop hits the ground, kill everyone on the spot, except for this one," the large man ordered, indicating Frenchie. "I want her to die real slow. Start with her arms and legs."

"Give it back to me, Dean, or you're all dead," Helen said quietly. "I couldn't stop them if I tried."

"They wouldn't shoot, because then I would drop your little 'children' all over the floor, and that would ruin your 'Final Crusade,'" Dean said, forcing an air of defiance. Inwardly, he was in anguish that his moment of absolute supremacy had passed.

"And we'll just do it again in a few months," Helen said calmly. "You can't stop us. No one can."

"Miller, pour the rest of it on the ground!" Tannenbaum demanded. "There won't be any second chances and they know it, they've lost their cover and their surprise. Do what you set out to do!"

"Dean, don't make us kill you," Helen said. "It's not worth it. Give that vial back. I promise, no hard feelings. One day, you'll rejoice that you did. Spill it, and you've condemned yourself, your friends and the world to death."

"Archers, prepare to shoot," Mr. Natural commanded.

"Miller, smash it!" Tannenbaum shouted.

"Why such an extreme plot, Helen?" Dean asked hesitantly. "Do billions of people really have to die just to save a bunch of trees?"

"This conversation would have been more relevant fifty years ago,"

Helen shot back. "The world is beyond the tinkering stage. Do you actually think for a moment that things will improve? Come on, they're getting worse by the minute! Dean, wake up, it's over. In some places you have to drive for hours just to see a tree. The only wild animals left are in the zoos, and yes, oh yes, Carol, lions and tigers are very sacred to me."

She whirled around to face the group, looking from one to the other.

"Everyone, now, think of beautiful things! Beaches, forest, vast meadows. You name it, and they're threatened. Now think of your favorite time period. Go ahead!"

Everyone stared at her, mesmerized by her intensity.

"I bet no one picked yesterday," she taunted. "Finkel, you're into the Greeks and Romans, right? Seen any of them lately? They don't exist anymore, do they, they're just in books. If they came back tomorrow they'd think they were on another planet. Big chief Tannenbaum, you're even worse. I know for a fact that your passion in life, besides running an ER department and killing little children, is ancient Egypt. Very relevant, I must say. Carol, what's your favorite?"

"I always liked the Victorians," she said numbly.

"Me too, did you know that? I loved their clothes, their manners, their elegance. A beautiful era. And you know what? They're all dead. Their time was long gone before your grandparents were even born.

"Ehler, you're into colonial times. I always found that so charming. So tell me, how many pilgrims have you seen lately?"

Helen turned to Frenchie.

"And you, my dear, what's your favorite? No cheating now, no answers like, 'in the future, with my beloved.' Tell me."

"The Middle Ages, I guess," Frenchie answered, her eyes on Dean. "I always wanted to be a lady, and live in a castle."

"Ahh, how lovely. What's the matter, everyone, how come no one picked this century?" Helen hissed, looking around. "You have something against subways or slums?

"Don't you see?" she shouted, punching the air with her fist, her voice almost a shriek. "The modern age is a high tech sham! The things you really love about the world are long gone. They're dead! We see movies about cowboys and kings, and we think they're real. They're not! They don't exist anymore, except in our minds. Half the world is already too dangerous to even visit. It's all going down the drain, and we don't recognize it because we're too busy worshipping the past!"

"You're sick," Tannenbaum snapped. "You have no right to hurt anyone. You're as evil as any blood thirsty dictator who's ever lived."

"Like I said, I took the right to do this," Helen said. She turned and walked up to Dean. Her face was within inches of his. He didn't move. "Dean, give me the beaker. Save yourself and your friends."

"This isn't happening," Dean moaned, his face twisted with anguish. "You're asking me to help you destroy the world."

"Do we have to kill someone to demonstrate that we're serious?" Helen asked, not taking her eyes off of him. "Natural, kill Frenchie at the count of three."

Two warriors walked up and stood over Frenchie. They pulled their bows taut and aimed directly at her face. She flinched but didn't look away.

"You wouldn't dare!" Dean gasped.

"We'll be killing all of them except you, Dean," Helen whispered, her lips pulled back, her eyes bulging. "You'll have this great big world all to yourself. You and your six billion friends."

"Please …"

"One!"

"Helen, don't make me choose."

"Then you should have stayed out of this. It's your decision, Dean, not mine. What'll it be, the world you love, or the world gone mad?"

"I can't."

"Two!"

"Helen, wait, please. Fink, what should I do?"

"Go ahead, Bob, tell him," Helen said. Her eyes continued to bore into Dean's. "You know, this decision probably is too important just for you to make. So let's have a forum. Bob, talk to the good doctor."

"I don't want to die, Dean, and I don't want Carol to die," Finkel said, his voice trembling. "I just found a reason for living, and don't care all that much about anything else. Give the crap back to her."

"He's right, Dean," Carol implored. "Strangers aren't worth dying for. For twenty years I took care of people who would spit in my face. Maybe I'm just not that good a person, but, damn, I want to live so much now!"

"Don't listen to them, Miller," Tannenbaum shouted. "This is madness. Don't help them destroy the world."

"I agree with the chief," Ehler said in measured tones. "Dean, you deliberately chose to work in a place where the worst of humanity is on display, each and every day. It's a game we play, and yeah, we do it for the money. But it's gotten to you, you've become blind to the beauty in this world. I'm not worried about dying. Life must go on. Do *not* give it back to her, Dean. Hopefully, one day my kids will understand."

"Spoken like a true humanist," Helen said with quiet intensity. Her eyes burned into his. "I think we have a tie, Dean. Are you ready to cast the deciding vote? Let's restart the countdown."

Dean's mind was racing, as fragments of his life flew before him. Images of his childhood, his crumbled marraige, of him and Frenchie making love, of the stricken men in the courtyard, of the day's purple and orange sunset, they all blinded and confused him. The blue liquid in his hand seemed totally serene, impervious to the drama that it had inspired.

"Frenchie!" Dean cried out.

"Dean, I'm with you all the way, whatever you do. I'll always be with you!"

"One."

"Frenchie, will you marry me in heaven?" he shouted.

"Yes, a thousand times yes!" she screamed.

"What is the best way to die, Dean?" Helen asked gently. "'Saving the world', you once said. Well, here's your chance. *Two.*"

Dean looked at Toot on the rock. The man smiled at him peacefully. What's going to happen is going to happen, his eyes seemed to say.

Dean turned to Helen.

"Here," he said, and he gently passed the vial back to her.

"Thank you, Dean," she said softly.

Two warriors pushed Dean several feet away. Jungle Man walked over to the large vat and put his hands on the edge. Carefully, Helen poured the liquid into the mixture. A puff of blue steam wafted over the top. She then placed her hands on the other side of the cauldron.

"No!" Tannenbaum shouted. He shot to his feet, his hands still securely tied. He charged towards them, rage in his eyes. Three arrows whistled through the air and pierced his chest simultaneously. He crashed onto the floor in front of the vat, breathing heavily.

"Traitors!" he rasped, "You traitors …"

And then he lay still. Dean and the others stared at his body in horror.

Helen nodded at Jungle Man, and the two of them tilted the vat onto its side. The pale blue potion splashed loudly into the large pool of water. No one moved, their eyes riveted on the scene. Aside from the splashing sounds, the cavern was, for a moment, deathly still.

chapter 69

"Come look, if you like," Helen said excitedly, breaking the silence. "Dean, everyone, come take a look!"

Everyone in the room walked over to the edge of the water. Warriors lowered their bows that had been aimed at Dean and his friends as they too arose. Their fight was over.

The dark water was foamy with blue bubbles. It swirled and weaved around several rocks, and exited twenty feet away, into a wall. Dean knew that somewhere, one or more streams would emerge from this mountain and trickle onwards, eventually emptying into the small river that ran alongside the park. The river, in turn, would eventually merge with others, and in a matter of days, reach the ocean. The process was now unstoppable.

The warriors all started to cheer and pound each other on the back. Mr. Natural let out a whoop and began dancing with joy. Dean sat down heavily, his eyes closed. Frenchie looked at him helplessly. Finkel, Carol and Ehler all seemed to be in shock. They stared dumbly at the water, which was starting to clear in front of their eyes.

Toot jumped off the rock and went over to Godfrey, who remained on the ground. Helen and Jungle Man hugged.

"My sweet Cassiana," he said affectionately.

Helen kissed his cheek. A second later, she turned to everyone. The room hushed.

"Listen, please, this is very important. The Final Crusade is complete. There will be time to celebrate later. But now, we must leave quickly. I doubt anyone heard all the commotion, but in the morning the bodies will be found. Proceed to the safe houses. Speak to no one, and take orders from your chief. In a few days you can all start your journey back to your home. Good-bye. I love all of you."

The men surrounded her, hugging and kissing her, some crying. Helen hugged and kissed them back.

"Come on, everyone, let's get to the vans," Mr. Natural said.

He looked at Helen, who had pulled away from the group.

"I'm heading to my cabin for a while. I'll see you at the village in Mexico, like we said. We'll watch the sky together, and look at the Southern Cross."

Helen smiled at him weakly. Mr. Natural turned and left.

The warriors began slowly filing out. Helen turned to Jungle Man, who stayed behind.

"I'll miss you," she said awkwardly.

"It does not have to be this way," he replied.

"I know where you'll be. We'll see."

"Maybe," he said sadly.

Jungle Man turned to Toot.

"Tuti, are you ready to come home?" he asked.

The man nodded, yes, I'm ready.

"Godfrey, you will come with us, right?"

"What about my sister," he mumbled through his swollen lips.

"She's fine. She had the protection."

"And she lives in Hawaii, no less. Talk about luck. Yes, I'll come with you."

Toot helped his friend slowly to his feet.

"Can you walk?" he asked Godfrey.

"Yeah, I'll be fine."

They turned to Dean. He remained seated on the floor by the pool, not moving.

"Good-bye, Doc, thanks for everything," Toot said, touching Dean's shoulder.

Dean didn't move.

"Tuti, it's time to go," Jungle Man said gently. "Meet us in the van."

As Toot turned to leave, Godfrey knelt down, wincing in pain, and spoke into Dean's ear.

"You're the hero, not me," he whispered. "Take good care of Frenchie."

Then, slowly, he straightened and walked out of the cavern with Toot.

Jungle Man gestured to Frenchie. "Why don't you go with them?" he asked.

"My place is with him," she said, looking at Dean, who remained motionless.

"Isn't that right, honey?" she asked him.

Dean didn't move. Frenchie looked at him with alarm.

After a few moments, Jungle Man spoke to her softly.

"Give him time," he said. "Come with us."

"Dean, don't you want me to wait with you?" she asked, her voice quivering.

With the barest of motions, Dean shook his head.

"Take me home," Frenchie finally said to Jungle Man. "I want to go home."

"Of course," the chief said. "We'll give you addresses and phone numbers if you need us."

"Dean, I'll be waiting for you," she pleaded, as she was gently led away. "I'll always be waiting for you. You said you were with me all the way. Call me."

Helen watched Jungle Man leave with Frenchie, and then stared at the lifeless body of Tannenbaum.

"He was to get the vaccine," she said, half to herself. "He was to be all alone in the world. That was my payback."

She turned to Finkel, Carol and Ehler.

"Follow the markers to the parking lot," Helen said, handing a paper and a set of keys to Finkel. "Your car is there. Go to this address. It's easy to find. Dan, your family is already there. There's plenty of money, and more than enough food. The numbers of the other houses are also listed.

"Listen, you're all covered, so no one suspects foul play. But my advice is, don't go back to the city. Stay out of sight for the next few days. What just took place is irreversible and should hit soon. If you tell anyone, you may be locked up for questioning, and you might literally die in custody. Take in a movie, go shopping, but keep a low profile. This isn't for my sake, it's for yours."

Finkel nodded at her, and put the paper in a pocket. He stared at a blue bubble floating among the small rocks below.

"This really was on the level, wasn't it," he murmured. "Is there any chance this is a nightmare, and that I'm going to wake up soon? Bad tacos or something?"

Helen smiled tightly and shook her head. Finkel nodded at her and smiled.

"In that case, I think it's time to load up on dental floss," he said, straightening up. "Come on guys, let's hit the road. Helen, what's going to happen to Dean? And you."

"I'll drive him to a safe house. He'll come around soon, he's tougher than he realizes. As for me, I'm going back to the city. I may even work a few shifts, so nobody suspects anything. It will also give me a chance to see what happens. Take good care, everyone. I don't think I'll ever be seeing you again."

She extended a hand. Ehler ignored it and walked out of the room, going through the opening in the wall and disappearing almost immediately. Carol shuffled uneasily, looking down. But Finkel took it, and they shook warmly.

"So, uh, who won, the good guys or the bad guys," he asked.

Helen smiled thinly and shrugged, almost imperceptibly.

"Good-bye, Fink."

Finkel dropped to a knee and hugged Dean. "I love you, guy," he whispered. "Call me when you're ready."

Dean nodded, his eyes still closed.

Gently, Finkel patted his friend on the shoulder, and stood up.

"Good-bye, Dean," Carol said. She leaned over and kissed him on the forehead.

The two of them left. Helen sat down next to Dean and looked into the water. They were alone.

A few minutes passed before Dean opened his eyes. He looked down and saw the water dancing amongst the rocks in the stream. One or two bluish bubbles remained, floating aimlessly on the surface. Together they sat in near silence, in the somber, torch lit cave. The walls gently echoed with the sounds of water.

Finally, Helen broke the silence

"How do you feel?"

"Like I'm drifting in cold, dark space," he said. "I feel like I'm dead."

"This was all my doing, you know," she said flatly. "I take all the responsibility, and I'll take all the fire hell has to offer, if that is the final judgment on me."

"Helen, why did you do it?" Dean asked in a whisper.

"I don't know exactly ~~know~~, but one day, something snapped. I sensed all this injustice, and knew I was meant to fight it. Things snowballed after that. Is that the reason you wanted?"

"Is that all?" he asked.

"No."

"Do you feel any better now?"

"No, all the pain is still there."

"Helen, take me out of here."

They both got up. Dean felt as if he was floating, and he had trouble feeling his legs. I am the walking dead, he thought.

As they were exiting the cave, Helen tapped on his shoulder. Dean turned to look at her, he noticed how deeply tired her face was, and how her eyes seemed to have lost their glow.

"I have something to tell you," she said.

"What is it?" he asked.

"I didn't take the vaccine. I figure I have about a week."

Dean wanted to be angry with her, for leaving him to feel all the pain and guilt alone, but nothing happened. Dead people have no emotions, he said to himself.

"It's time to go," he said.

chapter 70

Connigan lounged on a bed of grass, looking at the stars, drifting into sleep. The summer breeze almost felt sweet as it brushed past his face. Pony sat beside him, cradling his head in her lap, watching over him. Every minute or so she would bend over and kiss his lips and eyes, her breasts rubbing against his face. She tried not to awaken him, and he tried his best at pretending not to notice her kisses, which made her giggle. Both of them knew that soon, when he was rested, she would begin making passionate love with him.

His world was peaceful and joyous. Everywhere around them were the most delightful plants and animals—he could have sworn he had just seen a unicorn—and even other people, although they were few in number and maybe hundreds of miles away. Everyone knew that in paradise you respected other people's boundaries. There was more than enough for everyone.

"John," a voice called out from the bushes.

Connigan felt Pony stiffen protectively over him. As peaceful as she appeared, he knew she was a master at defense, and was more than capable of keeping him from danger.

"John, it's me," the voice said.

"Who are you?" he blurted out, sitting up.

Doctor X stepped out from behind the bushes.

Pony moved into an attack crouch, ready to leap. Connigan eyed the intruder suspiciously. The doctor backed up, holding up her hands.

"Easy there, easy there, Big John, I'll be gone in a minute," she said. "Listen to me, we're all done. We did it. Did you hear me? We did it, you and me. It's all over."

"You'll leave me alone now?" Connigan asked anxiously. The winds always blew icily when the doctor was around, and clouds would appear from nowhere. He touched Pony's muscular thighs for support. She reached out and held his hand, keeping her eyes on the stranger at all times.

Doctor X stared at the quaking man.

"Yes, John, I'm going, I'll leave you alone. Over here is a basket with food, enough for several days. There's also a plane ticket. Please do what we agreed on, and go on that trip. People will meet you as arranged, and take very good care of you. You'll have nothing to worry about."

The doctor nudged the basket toward Connigan. He recoiled from it.

"John, do you want to talk? Any words, any thoughts, anything about what we've done?"

"I just want you to leave me alone!"

"Catch that plane, don't forget. Take care, John. Your brilliance was awesome. You rescued the world."

With that the doctor eased herself backwards, and quietly blended into the darkness. As if by magic the stars brightened, and the trees and bushes came to life again.

"Do you think Doctor X is gone?" he asked nervously.

"Gone forever," Pony said, sitting down again. "You saved the world, John. You are, and always will be, my hero."

"And now, my love, I never have to leave you again. And I never will."

She leaned forward and tenderly kissed him, easing him onto the soft, warm ground. Drunk on their mutual passion, they merged into one, each nearly aching with joy.

Above them a large shooting star silently crossed overhead, celebrating the new age.

chapter 71

He didn't remember being driven to the safe house. When they stopped, he briefly came out of his fugue and looked around, wondering where they were. Then, seconds later, the numbing oblivion returned. Helen led him upstairs to a bedroom, and closed the door after him. Dean crashed into bed, fully clothed. Before sleep overwhelmed him he dimly heard her car racing off down the road.

There were no clocks and he had no idea of how long he had slept. Dean awakened feeling no less tired and he lay in bed, hour after hour, getting up only for the bathroom or to drink some water that had been left on the dresser.

Time ceased to matter, and he marked days only by the sunlight that would visit him with regularity. When it left he would lie in the dark room, staring into the night.

One night he decided to turn on the evening news, so that he could hear the pronouncement that the end had come. It's only right that it's announced on television, he thought. Otherwise it's not official.

A news show had just begun. The lead story detailed the outbreak of influenza, rare for the warm months. Both news anchors were out sick, and replacements were sitting in. I know something you don't know, he said to them in a singsong voice.

He decided to finally shower and shave. When he finished he returned to the bed and lay naked, staring at the ceiling. Maybe the whole thing was a dream, or maybe I'm dead and this is my hell, he thought.

He picked up the phone and called Helen.

He was not surprised that she was home.

"Yes?" she answered.

"It's me, Dean."

She was quiet for a few seconds.

"It's nice to hear your voice, Dean. The past few days ..."

"Was it a dream, Helen?"

"No, I'm sorry."

With an effort he forced himself to speak.

"So, how are you feeling?" he asked.

"Tired. That may be the first symptom, although it's a little early. It's very hard to predict this thing. We didn't have the luxury of long-term experimentation ..."

"How are things in the ER?" he asked.

"I never went back to work. It doesn't make any difference anymore. I'd just get depressed looking at all the people, you know, the ones I just ..."

"Helen, I feel so bad."

"Hang in there, Dean. The world needs you now. You'll be one of the pioneers, the founding fathers. You may be the one to preserve the written word, or the basic concepts of art and science. You've got to survive."

"Thanks for the assignment."

"Dean, I visited Frenchie."

"You did what?" he asked, sitting up in the bed.

"I almost got killed going to her place, but I had to tell her you were all right. She gave me a note for you. I had someone on the caravan slip it under your door when they were driving past your area. Frenchie didn't want to go with them. She's sticking it out in the city."

"What caravan?"

"Jungle Man, Toot, Godfrey and all the men left yesterday for our southern house. They should be there by now. They wanted a good head start for the long trip back home. I really can't say that I blame them."

"What are you going to do?" he asked.

"Me, I'm just curled up in my room, reading a book, sipping some wine. Hey, I finally went ahead and bought the best there is. It's funny, after the second glass, it all tastes the same."

"What are you reading?"

There was a pause.

"It's not important. Dean, go outside soon and look at the heavens. We're in the middle of a meteor shower. I read about it in the papers. I'd see it myself but there's all this light pollution here in the city. Well, I guess I'll get off now. Is there anything else you want to say?"

Dean looked at the phone and shook his head. No, I guess not, he thought to himself. What would you like me to say, Helen? That I'll try my best not to hang myself from some tree? That I'll learn to live with what I've done? Why should I, you won't.

After a short while Helen broke the silence.

"Well, good-bye then. And now, I'm going to disconnect the phone. Good-bye, Dean. Good luck to you."

Dean hung up the phone and went to the closet. There were clothes of several different sizes, and he found a loose fitting, comfortable out-fit. Then he went downstairs and walked to the front door. There was a letter that had been slipped under it. He opened it and pulled out a small piece of paper, apparently Frenchie's personalized stationery. In the upper, corner, circled by pink roses, was a drawing of a small castle. He recognized her handwriting.

> *I gave you what I could.*
> *Time is all I have left,*
> *Tomorrow, my final gift.*

Dean folded the poem and tucked it into his pocket. Time to see the meteors, he thought.

He walked out of the house and found himself on an empty beach. It's Helen's beach house, he said to himself. I should have guessed.

The beach was deserted except for a few seagulls, who regarded him quizzically, as if asking, "What are you doing out here at night, on our beach?"

"Excuse me, but I came to see the light show," he said to them.

His answer appeared to satisfy their curiosity, because they casually flew away. Dean walked out onto the sand. He sat down and looked at the horizon.

Almost immediately, a shooting star flew before him. It was a bright one, and seemed to actually leave a trail as it fled into the distance and disappeared. He was caught off guard, and didn't have time to make a wish. Give me one more chance, he thought. Just one more.

He looked above, marveling at how tantalizingly close, yet forever distant, the heavens seemed. The stars seemed to beckon to be touched, appreciated, if only one knew how. There's a secret to all this, he thought, to everything, and I bet it's right in front of me. This world will go on. Maybe one day I'll make sense of it all. Dean smiled for the first time in what seemed ages, as Connigan's words came back to him—life is like Jupiter, it's a roller coaster ride through purple infinity.

Suddenly, two meteors shot through the sky. I'm ready for you now, he thought. He closed his eyes and wished. When he opened them, they were gone.

Dean sensed it was time to go back, and he returned to the house.

He went up to his room and sat on the edge of the bed. And from a small world, may a larger one grow, he thought. And now, it's time for the second wish.

He picked up the phone and dialed. Frenchie answered on the first ring.